101
SECRETS
of a High-Performance
Veterinary Practice

by Bob Levoy

Veterinary Medicine Publishing Group
Lenexa, Kansas

Dedicated with love to Martha and Lynn,
who are the sunshine of my life.

Printed in the United States of America
Library of Congress Catalog Card Number 96-060137
ISBN 0-935078-60-6

10 9 8
First printing: October 1996

Table of Contents

How to Find and Hire Top-Notch Employees

1. Identifying Desirable Traits
2. Wording the Classified Ad
3. Creative Ways to Recruit New Employees
4. Job Sharing
5. Beware of Pre-Programmed Job Applicants
6. Getting Beyond the Résumé
7. Uncovering an Applicant's Inner Traits
8. The Inside Story
9. How Likable is the Person You're about to Hire?
10. Hard-Learned Lessons about Hiring

Give Your Practice a Competitive Advantage

11. The Commodity Trap
12. Differentiate Your Practice
13. Secrets of Award-Winning Service
14. It Starts at the Top
15. The Expectations Gap
16. Catering to "Cat People"
17. Is Your Practice Feline Friendly?

Image Management

Market Research

Fee Strategies

Stress Management

Acknowledgments

I am indebted to many people for their ideas, insights, and inspiration. Among them:

- Countless veterinarians and staff members who've attended my seminars; provided invaluable feedback; allowed me to visit their practices, pick their brains, and talk with their clients; and who've shared their secrets of high-performance practice.
- Many corporate clients and seminar sponsors who've enabled me to spread the word about practice management and marketing to veterinary audiences throughout the world.
- The publishers and editorial staffs of *Veterinary Economics* magazine, past and present, for their encouragement and support from the start, and for providing a widely read forum for my monthly column, "Bob Levoy's Success File."
- Becky Turner, Editorial Director of Veterinary Medicine Publishing Group, for polishing and skillfully editing my manuscript.
- And most important, my wife, best friend, and editorial consultant, Martha Eagle Levoy, for her keen insights and constructive comments during the development of this book.

I thank you all.

How to Get the Most from this Book

How profitable was the last management book you read? Was it stimulating for the moment—and soon forgotten? Or was it the beginning of a journey of significant practice growth? The following suggestions are intended to help you wring more usable ideas from this book and greatly increase your return on investment.

Don't analyze the recipe; taste the cake. Think of the bumblebee. Nothing that flies is less qualified to do so. Its wings are undersized for its body; its overall configuration is awkward and unsuited for flight. Yet despite the laws of aerodynamics, the bumblebee defies the impossible. It flies.

Some of the ideas in this book operate on the same principle. On paper, they may not "seem" as if they'd work. Yet the people who are associated with these ideas can attest to their value.

After a recent seminar I conducted, a veterinarian wrote: "I must admit I was skeptical about the value of schematic drawings to help clients understand various conditions affecting their pet's health. It struck me as time-consuming and possibly a bit pushy. But about 10 days after the seminar, I happened to be talking with my internist about the results of my annual physical exam.

"During the discussion, he used a schematic drawing of the heart, and he narrowed the coronary arteries to illustrate the dire consequences of my high-cholesterol diet and lack of exercise. He then gave me the drawing and told me to tape it to my refrigerator door."

"As well as I know the subject," he continued, "the drawing made such an impact that not only have I gone on a diet, I've also started to make drawings for my clients—with excellent results in both cases."

The moral? *Non tentare, non pugnare.* (If you haven't tried it, don't knock it.)

Seek improvement, not perfection. Prospect for nuggets, not the whole lode. Don't limit yourself to ready-made gems of wisdom. Be on your toes to recognize how the ideas in this book can be *modified* to make them more valuable to your practice.

In the following pages, you'll find ideas that will start a chain reaction of thoughts and perhaps lead to an inspiration. This book may start such "spring-boarding"—but only you can finish with reflection and creative thinking.

Remember how little a pound of iron is worth until it is converted into horseshoes or needles or watch springs. By the same token, the more creatively you make use of what you read, the more profitable these ideas will be.

Don't be trapped by either-or thinking. It was Robert Benchley who quipped: "There are two kinds of people in the world: those who divide people into two kinds—and those who don't." That's either-or thinking. So is to say that what you read in this book must be implemented across the board, or not at all.

Take delegation, which is discussed in Chapter 6. Although delegation is a proven way to enhance a doctor's productivity and the job satisfaction of the staff member to whom a higher-level task is delegated, it's not for everyone. Some doctors prefer not to let go of the reins, and some staff members don't want the responsibility of taking them. In other words: Use the strategies in this book *selectively*.

Develop an action plan. I believe in defacing the books I read: underlining key passages, writing marginal notes, summarizing the highlights. Doing so has two purposes: First, it provides a memory device. As the proverb states, "the strongest memory is weaker than the palest ink." Second, the underlining and marginal notes provide a "decoding opportunity" to transform the author's words into a more personally meaningful and easily remembered form.

Take a chance on change. As the old saying goes, "If you keep on doing what you've always done, you'll keep on getting what you've always got." What you may be missing is a new way of doing things that's easier, more efficient, less stressful, or in some way better than the old way.

Embrace new ideas. Give new strategies and ways of doing things a chance to succeed. Some will work. Some won't. Next!

In the boardroom of a major corporation is a small sign that reads, "Nothing will ever be attempted if, first, every possible objection must be overcome."

Prologue

Every morning in Africa, a gazelle wakes up. It knows that it must run faster than the fastest lion or it will be killed. Every morning a lion wakes up. It knows it must outrun the slowest gazelle or it will starve to death. It doesn't matter whether you're a lion or a gazelle. When the sun comes up, you'd better be running.

> —From an article by Nancy Austin
> in the September 1995 issue of
> Working Woman *magazine*

This quotation captures the spirit of veterinary practice in today's highly competitive environment. The competition for clients, while perhaps not as predatory, is nonetheless intense and getting more so. Top-notch employees are hard to find and difficult to keep. Clients themselves are more discerning and demanding than ever before. And less loyal.

What's needed to build a high-performance practice in this environment? What are the secrets of keeping client satisfaction, practice growth, and employee productivity in high gear?

The first step: Get the right people on board.

1

How to Find and Hire Top-Notch Employees

Identifying Desirable Traits

1

Tip

The more compatible the new employee is with his or her co-workers, the better staff morale, motivation, and teamwork will be.

The first step in finding and hiring a great employee is to define "top-notch"—what skills, experience, and personality traits are you really looking for?

That question isn't as easy as it may seem. At the workshops I conduct on personnel management, I ask veterinarians and hospital managers to describe the ideal receptionist. The profiles vary from one practice to another —and sometimes from one individual to another in the same practice.

For valuable insights on the best type of person to hire for your practice, ask your staff this question: "If you could hire anyone for this job, what type of person would you look for?"

The next step: Review the following list of character traits, and add others of your own choosing. Select the five or so traits you consider most important. Doing so will greatly increase your chances of finding the person you seek.

ambitious	eager to learn	good listener
cheerful	empathetic	good self-esteem
common sense	energetic	hard-working
conscientious	enthusiastic	high tolerance
consistent	ethical	for contact
creative	flexible	honest
curious	focused	imaginative
detail-oriented	friendly	independent
diplomatic	goal-oriented	intelligent

kind
likable
likes challenges
loves animals
loyal
neat
organized
patient
possesses people
 skills
perceptive

persistent
personable
polite
proactive
productive
punctual
resourceful
respectful
responsible
self-motivated
sense of humor

sincere
stamina
team player
tenacious
thorough
time aware
warm
well-groomed
works well under
 pressure

From the Success File

Robert C. Brown, DVM, owner of the Cherrydale Veterinary Clinic in Arlington, Va., estimates that approximately 40 percent of the clients visiting his hospital are there only to purchase a prescription refill or over-the-counter product; drop off a urine or stool sample; or leave a pet. In most cases, they don't speak to a doctor or technician.

Dr. Brown views such transactions as opportunities for client education and for reinforcing the importance of "wellness care," which, according to Dr. Brown, " is the prevention of preventable diseases and conditions and the early detection and treatment of those that are not preventable."

Based on this philosophy, Dr. Brown looks for front-desk personnel with a background in teaching, preferably in elementary education. Two former teachers are on the staff now, both at salaries commensurate with their background.

Alternative Strategy

Circulate the list of traits to all staff members and ask each person to check the five traits he or she considers most important in a co-worker. Discuss the results at a staff meeting and reach a consensus. Doing so will expedite your search for the right person and establish standards for new and current staff members.

Wording the Classified Ad

Tip

Use words that describe the job in an appealing way; for instance: fast-growing, state-of-the-art practice; interesting and challenging work; friendly, caring environment; excellent salary/benefit package. Don't, however, promise more than you can realistically deliver.

How do you word a classified ad in order to attract top-notch applicants? Review your findings from Success Secret 1 and incorporate the traits you are looking for into your ad. For example:

We are looking for a warm, friendly individual who loves animals and has good people skills, a pleasant telephone voice, and the ability to handle a busy veterinary medical practice while maintaining a sense of humor. Computer skills are a plus.

From the Success File

The following is excerpted from a help-wanted ad for EuroDisney:

We need strong team players with:
- *exceptional people skills*
- *constant smiles*
- *never-say-no attitudes*
- *friendly, helpful, courteous demeanors.*

Creative Ways to Recruit New Employees

3

Finding top-notch employees who are hardworking, personable, dependable, able to leap tall buildings, and so on isn't easy in today's tight job market. If the usual recruiting channels aren't producing qualified candidates, consider the following:

- Offer a recruiting bonus of $100 to $200 to any staff member who recommends an individual who is later hired. In some cases, your current employees can publicize a job opening far better than a half-inch ad. Plus, if an employee you respect likes someone well enough to recommend him or her, the odds are better than average that the new person will fit in with your staff.
- If one of your *clients* possesses all of the traits you're looking for, consider recruiting him or her. You might ask: "I'd love to have someone with your personality working here. Do you know of anyone?" The person may be interested in the job—or know of a friend who might be. I know of many veterinary personnel who were hired in exactly this way.

Tip

At the outset, make it clear that the same high standards and selection process will be used to evaluate job applicants recommended by staff members. Stating this policy up front helps avoid any obligation you may feel to hire someone you don't consider the best choice for your practice.

Job Sharing

4

If you're unable to find qualified, full-time hospital personnel, consider *job-sharing,* which enables part-time employees to divide the work done by one full-time person. It also allows them time off for child care, elder care, schooling, or other responsibilities that prevent them from taking a full-time position.

The benefits of job-sharing include:

- the retention of skilled, enthusiastic, loyal personnel who have other part-time needs
- reduced absenteeism and turnover
- reduced overtime
- improved employee morale
- more peak-period coverage
- higher productivity

Best of all, there is a large and growing pool of highly qualified and motivated potential employees who are interested in part-time work.

Cost consideration: As a general rule, employers are not required under current law to provide fringe benefits for employees who work fewer than 1,000 hours a year.

Beware of Pre-Programmed Job Applicants

5

Have you ever hired someone who sounded great in the interview, then fell short on the job—even after extensive and expensive training? What went wrong?

In today's tight job market, job seekers are increasingly savvy. Among the reasons for this trend: a slew of "how to get the job you want" books. Applicants who do their homework are primed for the standard interview questions with well-prepared answers that may mislead you.

For example, if you ask, "Why have you changed jobs so frequently?" a clever applicant may tell you, "I moved as opportunities arose to broaden my experience. Now I want to settle down and utilize this diverse background in a job I really care about." Or if you ask, "What are your weaknesses?" he or she may say, "I tend to be a perfectionist."

Don't get me wrong. Such responses may be 100 percent legitimate. But experience shows that some applicants use programmed answers to deceive prospective employers and "get the job." And in these litigious times, even reference checks may fail to verify the accuracy of such information.

One way to protect yourself from such deception is to ask interview questions for which "good" answers are less obvious. For example, as an ice-breaker at the start of an interview, you might ask: "Tell me about the pets you've had." This question is more likely to evoke an honest, unrehearsed answer than the standard "tell me about yourself" question—which is almost always included in interview-preparation books.

From the Success File

Southwest Airlines is known for its always cheerful and helpful employees. Their secret? "We tend to hire people with empathy," explains Libby Sartain, the vice president of Southwest's People department. "We want to treat customers as individuals, not numbers on boarding passes. That's our sense of warmth.

"When we hire people, we ask them to give us an example from their previous jobs of how they treated a customer who had a problem and how they made it a win-win situation. And we hire only those people who can give us examples of how they treated customers the way we like them to be treated."

Getting Beyond the Résumé

Open-ended questions take you beyond the résumé, the hype, and pre-programmed answers. Such questions also allow job applicants to tell you more about themselves, and they allow you to make more informed hiring decisions.

Consider these tested interview questions the next time you meet with an applicant:

- What are you looking for in your next job that's missing from your present one?
- Do you prefer to work alone or with others?
- What about your work do you find most challenging?
- What aspects of your last job did you like best? Least?
- What job-related situations have you found most stressful?
- What have you found most effective in dealing with such stress?
- What do you consider your greatest strengths? Don't be modest.
- What benefits do you think pets bring to their owners' lives?
- How do you feel about animal euthanasia?
- In which of your jobs did you learn the most?
- Tell me about the best boss you ever had. What about the worst?
- Have you ever seen a veterinary technician/assistant/ receptionist (depending on the position for which you are hiring) show especially poor judgment? If so, please tell me about it.

6

Tip

For the best results, use only a few of the questions listed here and probe for further information with such follow-up requests as "please explain" or "that's interesting, tell me more."

7

Uncovering an Applicant's Inner Traits

Tip

As a final question, consider asking the job applicant: "Is there anything you'd like to discuss that we haven't talked about?" See if the person asks about job content, your expectations, why the last person left, or other related questions that may provide clues to his or her inner traits.

After considering job skill and experience, many veterinarians appraise job applicants according to appearance, personality, or their love of animals. While these are important traits, they aren't enough.

Far more important are a person's "inner traits": intelligence, inner drive, attitude toward work, and ability to get along with others. These factors determine whether a person with the right job skills and experience will be right for your practice. Here are some questions to help you assess your candidate's inner traits:

- In your last job, what accomplishments gave you the most satisfaction?
- In your last job, what did you do when you finished work ahead of schedule?
- Do you like a boss who gives you a lot of responsibility or one who provides a lot of supervision?
- Have you learned any new skills or explored a new field of interest—even a hobby—since leaving school?
- What experience have you had working in groups or with a team? Did you ever have to deal with a team member who didn't cooperate or contribute a fair share of the work? What did you do in those situations?

The Inside Story

8

Cleanliness, neatness, and attention to detail are important traits for most jobs in a veterinary hospital. The problem: How do you evaluate job applicants on such matters? Handwritten job applications and personal grooming are two ways. Here's another:

When interviewing potential associates and key personnel for the Harvester Animal Clinic, Inc., in St. Charles, Mo., Don Polley, DVM, takes each of the leading candidates to lunch. The informal discussion in a neutral setting puts the applicants at ease, encourages them to "open up," and often reveals something that is helpful in making a final decision.

Now to the inside story: For the short drive to the restaurant, Dr. Polley asks candidates to drive him in their own cars. The car's upkeep—or lack of it—can speak volumes about the hard-to-evaluate traits mentioned above. For example, interiors that are dirty and unkempt say one thing; those that are neat and clean say something entirely different. Sometimes the contents themselves or the smell of the car send messages that either confirm or contradict Dr. Polley's first impression of the job applicant.

To test this theory, check the interior of your own car. How accurately does it speak for you?

How Likable is the Person You're about to Hire?

9

Some staff members are personable and instantly likable; others are less so. And oh, what a difference it makes—in the rhythm and image of the practice, and in client satisfaction and referrals.

A likable personality is an asset—some say a necessity—in any service occupation, veterinary medicine included. But it's frequently underestimated—or completely overlooked during the hiring process.

What is a "likable personality"? Bobbie Gee, image consultant and author of *Creating a Million Dollar Image for Your Business* (PageMill Press, 1991) says likable people:

- smile easily
- have a good sense of humor
- are great listeners
- know common-sense etiquette and use it
- are self-confident
- engage you in conversation about yourself
- can laugh at themselves
- are approachable.

For a veterinary practice, I'd add that likable people are:

- patient
- empathetic
- people who *truly* like all kinds of pets and their owners.

Such personality traits can't be "faked." And written scripts are, for the most part, transparent. Even training, sad to say, is of little help. In other words, what you hire is essentially what you get.

When interviewing job applicants, pay special attention to their personalities. Do they have the above-mentioned traits or others you deem important? Are they easy to like? Ask current employees to judge the likableness of those you're thinking of hiring. Doing so will raise everyone's awareness of the "Likable Factor" and its importance to a successful practice.

Question: How likable are you? In his book, *Kids Don't Learn From People They Don't Like*, (Human Resources Development Press, 1977), author/educator David Aspy writes that when students don't like a teacher, they develop a resistance to learning. Students, it seems, do best with teachers they *like*.

My surveys indicate the same is true in the workplace. When employees like the veterinarians and hospital managers with whom they work, there tends to be less absenteeism and turnover, better morale and motivation, and more teamwork and productivity. And they speak openly about how much they love their jobs.

Take another look at the personality traits on the previous page. Knowing how well you rate may help improve the employee relations and esprit de corps of your practice.

10

Hard-Learned Lessons about Hiring

- If a new employee doesn't have the right work attitude or the right personality for your practice, it's unlikely on-the-job training will make a difference. Remember: Your practice is only as strong as the weakest employee.
- To compromise your standards because of a small applicant pool or because you're desperate is what I call the "buy now—pay later" approach to hiring.
- Beware of the "Halo Effect": being so dazzled by a quality in an applicant (e.g., appearance, friendliness, office skills) that you lose sight of other job requirements.
- Beware of a history of "job hopping." Three jobs in five years may be too many, unless the changes show a sensible pattern, such as higher pay or more responsibility.
- Beware of applicants who gossip about former employers, practices, or clients. You'll be next.
- Wanting to hire a highly qualified applicant may lead you to make promises you can't keep or that will anger other employees. Action step: Stick to written job descriptions.
- Allow employees to interview applicants and narrow the list from which you'll make the final decision. Or give them the final approval of someone you've tentatively decided to hire. Employees will get along better and show more team spirit if they have a voice in hiring decisions.
- Never hire someone whose first question is: "What are the benefits?" And never hire someone you can't fire, such as friends and relatives.

2

Give Your Practice a Competitive Advantage

The Commodity Trap

Reality Check

It's somewhat controversial, but it is done: "mystery" shopping the competition. One East Coast veterinarian, for example, pays staff members to visit other area hospitals to obtain treatment for their pets. Such visits can be extremely uplifting or depressing— depending on how your practice compares with others.

No doubt about it. Low-cost spay and vaccination facilities lure away significant numbers of clients from some practices. Our research indicates that many of these transfer clients believe veterinary medicine is a "commodity"—that is, a service that is standard in all respects, regardless of who provides it. To them, a spay is a spay—so why not have it done as inexpensively as possible?

My question to veterinarians caught in this bind: What differentiates your practice in a meaningful way from those to which your clients are switching? Many don't have an answer, and this lack of differentiation causes a vicious cycle: Clients are influenced by fees because they don't perceive a difference between one practice and another. Veterinarians, believing such clients to be strictly "price driven," fail to address the "commodity" image of their practices. The prophecy fulfills itself.

What's the solution? It's twofold, and you'll find strategies for both steps throughout this book.

Step 1. Determine the strengths and weaknesses of low-cost facilities and compare them with the strengths and weaknesses of your practice.

Step 2. Make sure your practice's competitive advantages offset the strengths of those practices, and that your practice is well-differentiated in your clients' eyes. Those who fail to take these steps are in danger of losing clients to low-cost facilities—especially in a down economy.

Differentiate Your Practice

12

One way to avoid the commodity trap and gain a potent, competitive advantage is to *differentiate* your practice. How? By making sure that something about it sets it apart from others in what Professor Michael Porter of Harvard University calls "substantial and sustainable" ways.

Among the many possibilities:

- Specialty board certification;
- A specialist on staff, part-time or otherwise;
- A limited practice such as feline or house-call;
- Clinical excellence;
- Outstanding service;
- State-of-the-art equipment;
- An in-house lab;
- Accreditation by the American Animal Hospital Association;
- A design award from *Veterinary Economics'* Hospital Design Competition;
- Extended hours;
- Operational efficiency (a well-run, on-time practice);
- A unique service such as 24-hour operation with a doctor on duty at all times, or other special services discussed in this chapter.

Continued

From the Success File

While in private practice, Clayton MacKay, DVM, director of the teaching hospital at the University of Guelph, Ontario, Canada, and the 1996 President of the American Animal Hospital Association (AAHA), took a special interest in behavioral management services. He offered in-office and house-call consultations at fees ranging from $80 to $150 an hour. Among the benefits to his practice:

- *highly appreciative clients (50 percent of the questions clients ask involve pet behavior);*
- *frequent media appearances on radio, TV, and in the newspaper—which led to heightened public interest and client inquiries;*
- *numerous referrals from other veterinarians unable to provide such services to their clients;*
- *the satisfaction of providing a much-needed service. (Consider this grim statistic: Forty percent of the people who own a dog are considering getting rid of it because of behavior problems.)*

Also from the Success File

William Allen Rood, DVM, JD, and William Thomas Riddle, DVM, co-owners of the Rood & Riddle Equine Hospital in Lexington, Ky., are surrounded by approximately 125 equine practitioners—all vying for essentially the same clientele. Yet 75 to 80 percent of the cases seen at their hospital are referred by colleagues. The reason? Specialization.

Among the 19 doctors on staff are two certified by the

American College of Veterinary Surgeons, and two certified by the American College of Veterinary Internal Medicine. One of the latter doctors also specializes in cardiology.

In addition, Drs. Rood and Riddle's state-of-the-art hospital, which is capable of meeting any horse's medical needs, includes such features as:

- *gamma camera for performing nuclear scintigraphy*
- *video endoscope*
- *diagnostic ultrasound*
- *neonatal intensive care*
- *the ability to digitize radiographs for computer enhancement.*

13

Secrets of Award-Winning Service

In 1992, the Ritz-Carlton became the first hotel chain to win the prestigious Malcolm Baldridge National Quality Award, which was established by Congress in 1987 to promote quality management. According to Owen Dorsey, vice president of human resources, corporate management didn't earn the award; the hotels' 10,000 employees did.

A three-day orientation introduces every Ritz-Carlton employee to the following fundamentals:

1. "Ritz-Carlton Hotel is a place where the genuine care and comfort of our guests is our highest mission."
2. "At the Ritz-Carlton, we are ladies and gentlemen serving ladies and gentlemen."
3. "The three steps of service expected of every employee are a warm and sincere greeting using the guest's name; anticipation and compliance with guests' needs; and a fond farewell."

Ritz-Carlton trains employees with a thorough orientation followed by on-the-job training, then job certification. Among the Ritz-Carlton training basics:

- Create a positive work environment.
- Practice "team-work" and "lateral service."
- React quickly to correct any problem immediately.
- Move heaven and earth to satisfy a guest.

- Smile—we are on stage.
- Assume responsibility for uncompromising levels of cleanliness.
- Use the proper vocabulary with our guests (words like "good morning," "certainly," "I'll be happy to," and "my pleasure").
- Always maintain positive eye contact.
- Be an ambassador of your hotel in and outside of the workplace.
- Always talk positively.

These award-winning fundamentals are good beginnings for veterinary practices striving to achieve client satisfaction.

It Starts at the Top

14

In his book, *The Will To Manage* (McGraw Hill, 1966), Marvin Bower says it is a manager's responsibility to spell out for employees "the way we do things around here." Bower's implied assumption is that unless you tell people what you want them to do and how you want them to do it, you have no right to expect them to infer by some mysterious means just what you have in mind.

From the Success File

The following letter, sent to a new employee of a physician's office, illustrates the principle Bower describes above.

Dear Chris,

Welcome aboard. We are pleased to welcome you to our healthcare team and want you to be part of our continued success. To that end, I want to take a minute to reiterate the reason for our being here. If you remember these principles, I guarantee you'll succeed at your job and reap the rewards. Remember:

- *Above all, you are here to serve patients. Each of us is. The patient signs our paycheck.*
- *Our practice is built on medical quality and patient service. Strive for uncompromising quality in every phase of your job. Efficiency, precision, and attention to detail are all part of serving the patient.*

- *Every person who walks through our door—patient, postman, management consultant, sales rep—is an honored guest. Each of us is an ambassador of goodwill. We want you to astonish them with your courtesy, concern, and genuine caring for their comfort and well-being.*
- *Know your patients. Greet them by name, with a smile, as soon as they walk in our door. Let them know you appreciate them.*
- *Handle any patient problems or complaints with the utmost courtesy, concern, and respect. Remember, the patient is our boss.*

In short, we are all working for the same goals. If we apply these principles of patient satisfaction and professional excellence to our particular skills every day, there's no stopping us. Again, I welcome you to our office and look forward to working with you for a long and rewarding future.

Sincerely,

The Expectations Gap

Reality Check

Idexx Laboratories Inc., of Westbrook, Maine, learned the following through a survey of 406 randomly selected pet owners throughout the United States:
• 61 percent expect a sick pet's blood-test results within 12 hours;
• 37 percent expect results while they wait at the hospital or clinic.

What percentage of your clients account for 75 percent of your referrals? Our studies indicate that in the typical practice, the answer is about 15 to 20 percent. Why so few? The answer lies in what I call "the expectations gap," or the disparity between clients' expectations about a visit to your hospital and their perception of the experience itself. Consider these three groups of clients:

1. Clients whose experience is essentially what they expected in terms of the quality of care, the service, the hospital environment, and so on. These clients are satisfied but give no further thought to their experience, one way or the other. As a referral source, they are members of the "silent majority."

2. Clients whose experience *falls short* of their expectations and who are disappointed with the care their pet received, the service they received, or some other aspect of their hospital visit. These clients are *dissatisfied* and may complain about fees, bad-mouth the practice, or even leave, depending on the severity of their expectations gap.

3. Clients whose experience *exceeds* their expectations and who are delighted by everything. These clients are more than satisfied—they're *enthusiastic.* In the typical practice, they represent the 15 to 20 percent of clients who account for 75 percent of the referrals.

Can you imagine what would happen if you and your staff could exceed the expectations of *another* 15 to 20 percent of clients and add them to your referral base? Your practice would be *inundated* with new clients!

Catering to "Cat People"

16

Cat owners are known for their high expectations. They expect everyone in the hospital to like cats and to understand their nature. What's surprising is how frequently veterinarians overlook this essential requirement when hiring new employees. It's no wonder clients complain that "they didn't seem to like cats," or "they treated my cat like an 11-pound dog." In many cases, they seek "a veterinarian who just sees cats."

To screen job applicants, Karen Preston, CVPM, hospital manager of All Cats Hospital in Largo, Fla., asks the following questions:

- What do you think it takes to be a top-quality veterinary practice?
- What interests you about a position in a feline practice? (The answer of an applicant Preston just hired: "I love cats and I love 'cat people.' ")
- Have you ever spent time in an environment with a cat?
- Do you have any allergies to cats?
- How do you think cats benefit their owners' lives?
- What do you like the most about cats? What do you like least?

Preston warns, "It's a bad sign if a job applicant hesitates or has no answer to such questions—possibly indicating that he or she doesn't recognize the importance of a pet in a person's life."

Continued

In screening applicants, Preston also looks for the following qualities:

- A sensitivity to the human/feline bond
- Respect for the natural behavior patterns and personalities of cats (e.g., independence, individuality, curiosity).
- The ability and the desire to be supportive of clients *and* cats, regardless of the circumstances—to share the joy of kittens; comfort a grieving client who's lost a beloved companion; deal humanely and effectively with an unruly cat; and so on.
- The willingness to make every client's visit a positive experience.

Hospital personnel with these qualities greatly increase the satisfaction and referrals of "cat people."

The Obvious Secret

David H. Spearman, DVM, of Easley, S.C., whose practice went from 20 to 50 percent feline in three years, explains the increase by saying: "You and your staff have to genuinely like cats. You can't fool cats. And you can't fool 'cat people.'"

Is Your Practice Feline Friendly?

A veterinarian told me about the feline-only practice that recently opened a couple of miles from his companion animal practice. "My staff and I," he told me, "have now become *very* feline friendly—including setting aside one afternoon a week for feline appointments only." Other ways to let clients know your practice is feline friendly:

- design separate entrances and/or reception areas for dogs and cats
- select a feline hospital mascot
- post photos of staff members holding cats
- wallpaper an exam room with a feline motif.

From the Success File

Alice Johns, DVM, owner of The Cat Doctor in Indianapolis, Ind., gives patients colorful catnip mice that she crochets while talking on the phone, attending meetings, or traveling. (She calls it her "productive fidgeting.") For kittens, Dr. Johns crochets smaller mice without catnip—called "lite mice." Needless to say, the crocheted cats are a big hit—with cats and clients.

In a more serious and substantial way, Dr. Johns has differentiated her practice by becoming board-certified in feline practice by the American Board of Veterinary Practitioners. At the time of this writing, she's one of only 22 veterinarians in North America who have achieved this designation.

Who's Number One in Your Practice?

18

Where do your practice's veterinarians and staff members park their cars? In the choice spots by the entrance of the hospital? Or are those reserved for clients?

The sales of a (nameless) dog food company were slipping—badly. The vice president of sales called a meeting and asked the group: "Which dog food is the most nutritious?"

"Ours!" shouted the group.

"Which company has the best advertising?"

"We do!" they said.

"Who has the best sales force in the industry?"

"We do!"

"If our dog food is the most nutritious, and if we've got the best advertising and the greatest sales force, then *why aren't we selling more dog food?*"

There was complete silence. Then, from the back of the room, a voice answered: "Because the damn dogs don't like the stuff!"

In pursuit of new clients, higher client transaction charges, and practice growth, veterinarians are sometimes more concerned with *their* needs and preferences than those of their clients. And like the dog food company, they're often the last to realize it.

If you've got top-notch skills and a state-of-the-art hospital but "business" isn't as good as it should be, take another look at:

- your communication skills
- the quantity and quality of time spent with clients
- your hospital's policies

- your fees
- your appointment scheduling
- the caliber of your staff
- and all the peripherals associated with client services.

Are these parts of your practice geared to your needs and preferences—or to those of your clients? Who is *really* number one in your practice?

From the Success File

Joyce M. Hansen RN, practice manager of the Northampton Veterinary Clinic in Northampton, Mass., puts the whole subject into proper perspective by saying, "Clients do us a favor by deciding to come to us—not the other way around."

Drive-Up Service

Drs. John E. Fountain, Richard F. Hill, and Don Pyle know that in today's fast-paced, time-pressured society, everyone is in a hurry. That's why they installed a drive-up window in their Animal Health Center, a mixed animal practice in Crestview, Fla.

The window is used primarily for dispensing, and it enables clients to complete transactions quickly and easily without leaving their cars. When clients want to pick up a prescription or retail item, pay a bill, or drop off a stool sample, they simply drive to the window, which is visible to the receptionist, and sound their horns for service. If they phoned ahead for an item, it's ready for them.

The window is most heavily used between noon and 2 p.m. on weekdays, and on Saturday mornings. "Clients love the service and convenience," Dr. Fountain says, "especially on a rainy day." Dr. Fountain recommends an awning or overhang at the drive-up window for just such occasions.

Language Fluency

A Queens, N.Y., practitioner, recognizing the growing Hispanic population in his area, made his receptionist the following offer: If she would take an adult education course in conversational Spanish, he would gladly pay her tuition—125 percent of it if she received an "A"—and upon completion, give her a raise. She accepted, completed the course (with an "A"), and got a raise. The doctor, in turn, now sees an increasing number of Hispanic clients.

If the numbers in your community justify it, consider hiring a bilingual associate or assistant. He or she will attract many non-English-speaking clients and perhaps referrals from colleagues unable to converse with such pet owners.

If that's not feasible, there's a do-it-yourself alternative: Audio-Forum offers 275 audio-cassette courses for 96 different languages. These vary in length from 1.5 hours (key phrases and vocabulary only) to 15 to 20 hours of recorded material. For a catalog, write or call: Audio-Forum, 96 Broad Street, Guilford, CT 06437; (800) 243-1234; in Connecticut, (203) 453-9794.

Even a few phrases clumsily said will make non-English-speaking clients smile—and feel less self-conscious about their limited English.

20

Reality Check

Did you know that 11 percent of the U.S. population speaks a language other than English at home—and the numbers are increasing? If you or your staff are unable to converse with the people in your community who speak little or no English, your practice is at a disadvantage—especially if other practices employ multi-lingual personnel.

21

Providing Gold Star Service for VIPs

Here's a simple, people-pleasing, pet-pleasing, income-producing idea for veterinary facilities that offer boarding services: When pets are brought in for boarding at the Manassas Animal Hospital in Manassas, Va., their owners choose between basic boarding and "Gold Star" services, which are "especially recommended for puppies and kittens, older animals, and those pets who may particularly miss their owners."

Gold Star services are described in a brochure as well as on a placard at the reception desk that reads:

> For owners who prefer more individual care of their pets, we offer VIP GOLD STAR SERVICE for an additional fee of $2.50 per day for cats, and $3.95 per day for dogs.

For cats, VIP service includes daily play in the greenhouse jungle gym, a complimentary nail trim, a bedtime snack, and individual attention. Gold Star dogs enjoy individual walk-and-play twice a day with an attendant, daily brushing, and a bedtime snack. If they stay more than five days, they also receive a complimentary nail trim and a beauty bath.

Do clients like it? Sharon Crawford, the hospital's receptionist, says that 75 percent of their boarding clients opt for the Gold Star service, noting that the savings on nail trims and baths alone are worth it for longer stays. "It really sells itself," Crawford adds, "and not just to upscale clients."

John M. Todd, DVM, founder of the six-doctor hospital, gives his wife Carol Todd, CVPM, credit for Gold Star boarding. "What we've found," he says, "is that clients truly appreciate the options they're given when boarding their pets. But to make it work," he cautions, "you have to deliver the services you say you will. And then some."

"You know the staff's efforts are appreciated," Dr. Todd adds, "when clients return for future boarding services and you see pets wagging their tails with excitement—and happy to be at our facility again."

Follow-Up Calls

22

This simple telephone call communicates your concern for clients and patients in unmistakable terms, and it helps differentiate your practice from high-volume, impersonal operations. It may even prove to be clinically significant.

It's the call you make the day after you castrate a horse or do a bovine cesarean section—just to "touch base" and see how the patient is doing. Or it's the call to clients after they visit with seriously ill or injured pets. These owners are likely to be so distraught at the time of the visit that they don't listen to your explanations or home-care instructions. Many are too distracted to think of the questions that occur to them later.

Some veterinarians assume worried clients will call them. And some do. But experience shows that many clients won't call because they don't want to disturb you.

To keep the calls short, preface them by saying you're between appointments, at home, or on your way home. Clients will realize that your time is limited.

Don't be surprised when these clients say, "I wish *my own doctor* took such interest."

A Pet Visitation Room

My company's research shows that a "no visitation" policy for hospitalized pets troubles many clients—from mildly to profoundly. These clients may switch to a practice more in tune with their needs, especially if the human hospitals in the area have relaxed their previously rigid rules—as many have today.

To meet clients' need to see their pets, the Morningside Animal Clinic in Scarborough, Ontario, not only allows visitation (medical condition permitting) but also provides a visitation room expressly for that purpose. Practice owner Avery Gillick, DVM, says the policy benefits pets, owners, and even the clinic's staff members.

According to Dr. Gillick, about 75 percent of the practice's clients with pets hospitalized for an extended stay visit their pets for an average of 5 to 15 minutes. A few clients spend considerably more time, and that too, is allowed. During such visits, staff members meet and talk with the clients, an opportunity that makes their work more interesting and enjoyable and that boosts their morale and motivation. "Staff members work with a lot more dedication if they know each other," Dr. Gillick says.

For the maximum utilization of the space, Dr. Gillick suggests giving a visitation room multiple purposes such as hospital discharges and extended client consultations.

Pick-Up/Drop-Off Service

24

My definition of marketing is simple: Find out what clients want—and give it to them. Marketing is *needs satisfaction*. If you can meet a client's unique needs and be the only practice in your area to do it, you've got a sure-fire formula for practice growth.

Dr. Kenneth Rotondo puts this concept to work by providing a pet pick-up/drop-off service for clients who live within an eight- to 10-mile radius of his hospital in Clifton Park, N.Y. He offers this door-to-door service from 7 a.m. to 9 a.m. and from 3 p.m. to 5 p.m. To make the rounds, a ward attendant drives a minivan equipped with four airline pet carriers. The fee: $20.

Dr. Rotondo says he receives 15 to 20 requests a week, most often from senior citizens with no means of transportation, and from dual-income families who put a premium on time. His one caveat: Check with your insurance carrier to make sure your policy provides proper coverage.

From the Success File

Another example of a unique pick-up service is the equine ambulance *provided by the Northwest Animal Clinic and Hospital in Albuquerque, N.M., which is owned by Michael Riegger, DVM. This converted, completely rebuilt horse trailer interfaces with his hospital's equine O.R. and can transport traumatized, injured, or seriously ill horses to his facility. "It's frequently requested by other veterinarians," says Dr. Riegger, "and has been great for referrals."*

Peace of Mind
for Troubled Clients

What can you do for terminally ill clients who live alone and are worried about what will happen to their pets when they no longer can care for them? Faced three times with this sad situation, AHT Melissa Fuller, who works for Dr. Greg Dye at the Green Oaks/Arkansas Animal Hospital in North Arlington, Texas, found a way to help.

Fuller suggests waiting until clients bring up the subject of what will happen to their pets when they're gone and only then gently inquiring: "Do you have any wishes concerning your pet that I can be of help with?"

To comfort these pet owners, Fuller and others on the staff help find new homes for the animals. They also feed and care for the pets—at no charge—until new owners can be found.

"It's worth the time and expense," Fuller says, "because it enables terminally ill clients to meet their pets' new owners. They have the chance to say 'good-bye' and to know their pets will be loved and taken care of. This knowledge gives them great peace of mind."

There are many components to a high-performance practice; two of them are empathy and kindness, as exemplified by the thoughtful staff of this hospital.

26

These Special Touches Say "We Care"

Tip

Another "we care" item that pleases clients at many veterinary hospitals: heated water pads under pets during surgery and recovery.

"Familiar objects are important in helping patients feel more relaxed and at ease in a strange environment," says Mary Grace Connolly, assistant professor at the Loyola School of Nursing. She suggests that family members bring patients such personal possessions as photos or stuffed animals to help provide a feeling of familiarity, comfort, and continuity with the outside world.

Encouraging such home-to-hospital continuity can be a strong *client* relations tool for veterinarians. William R. Roberson, DVM, in Little Rock, Ark., informs his clients:

> *We care about our patients and attempt to make their visits with us as comfortable as possible. If there is any item, such as a favorite blanket or toy with which your pet feels secure, please feel free to bring it with you.*

"Be extra careful with such toys because of the sentimental attachment," Dr. Roberson cautions. A small container by each compartment will provide safe-keeping during the cleaning process.

If a client doesn't bring a toy, the hospital provides one. Dr. Roberson says the response is positive. Allowing clients to provide familiar objects for their pets conveys a "we care" attitude that clients—and patients—greatly appreciate.

Making Your Practice Accessible to the Deaf or Hearing-Impaired

There are an estimated 20 million Americans who are hearing impaired, and two million who are deaf. Many are pet owners.

Chris Crosley, DVM, owner of the Riegel Animal Hospital in St. Louis, Mo., is making a special effort to address the needs of these clients. She and her staff recognize the special role companion animals play in the lives of their hearing-impaired owners and gladly give these clients the extra time that is sometimes needed.

In addition, the hospital is equipped with a TDD (Telecommunications Device for the Deaf), a typewriter-like device that attaches easily to any standard telephone and enables the hearing-impaired to communicate with the hospital via telephone-transmitted, typed messages displayed on a screen. (The cost: $250 to $500).

Dr. Crosley also knows ASL (American Sign Language), which allows her to communicate directly without handwritten notes, an interpreter, or a client's ability to read lips. (Only about 30 percent of spoken English can be understood by lip reading). In addition, she's involved with the hearing-impaired community through her work with various organizations. Dr. Crosley now has a loyal and increasing base of hearing-impaired clients.

For more information on how to make your hospital

Alert your receptionist to the possibility of receiving a call that typically begins: "This is the Relay Service. I have a relay call for your hospital ... " Telephone company personnel report that many receptionists hang up when they receive calls for the first time, thinking it's a sales pitch.

accessible to the hearing impaired, contact:

- Telecommunications for the Deaf Inc. (8719 Colesville Road, Suite 300, Silver Spring, MD 20910; 301-589-3786). This private, non-profit organization offers a list of vendors who provide products and services for the hearing impaired. The organization also publishes an international directory of TDD numbers, including professional practices. A one-year listing is $30.
- AT&T Accessible Communication Products Center (5 Woodhollow Road, Room 1-119, Parsippany, NJ 07054; 800-233-1222) offers TDDs and such related products as flashing light signaling devices.
- Gallaudet University Press (800 Florida Ave., NE, Washington, DC 20002-3695; 800-451-1073) offers a catalog of books and educational materials pertaining to hearing, speech, and vision impairment.
- Telecommunication Relay Services and Operator Services for the Deaf and Hard of Hearing. Offered by many phone companies, this service enables deaf, hard of hearing, or speech disabled people wishing to make a phone call to type their message on a TDD to reach a no-charge Relay Service operator who then relays the message to the party being called. The operator then relays the hearing person's reply by typing it back to the TDD user. (Directory Assistance can provide TDD users with the toll-free number of the Telecommunication Relay Service in your area.)

Home Euthanasia

Fifteen to 20 times each year, Stephen A. Brammeier, DVM, owner of the Kingsbury Animal Hospital in St. Louis, Mo., provides a service for clients with elderly and terminally ill pets that relatively few veterinarians offer: home euthanasia.

Dr. Brammeier says that home euthanasia is one of the most emotionally satisfying services he performs. Among the reasons: The pets are more comfortable in familiar surroundings, and there is less trauma for both pet and owner. What's more, clients feel freer to express their sadness—and there's no need to collect themselves before driving home.

"Euthanasia at home is perceived by many clients to be more 'natural' than when it is done at the hospital," Dr. Brammeier says. "It also removes the stigma associated with a client's last visit to the practice." In addition to his standard charges for euthanasia and disposal, Dr. Brammeier charges $60.25 for such a housecall, and a technician accompanies him to the client's home.

Pet owners are profoundly appreciative of the privacy afforded by home euthanasia, and they've referred others to Dr. Brammeier for this kind service.

Helping Children with Pet Loss

29

Reality Check

A study conducted by the American Animal Hospital Association (AAHA) reveals that 40 percent of clients who switch veterinarians do so due to dissatisfaction with the circumstances surrounding the death/euthanasia of their pet.

Many parents aren't sure how best to explain the death of a beloved pet to a child. With the best of intentions, some say the wrong thing, and sadly, create additional psychological problems for the child.

In their excellent book, *Pet Loss: A Thoughtful Guide For Adults and Children,* Herbert Nieburg and Arlene Fischer offer an entire chapter on helping children with pet loss, including a list of do's and don'ts that you may want to pass along to concerned parents. Among them:

- **Don't** say: "The pet ran away and won't be coming back." Doing so may cause the child to feel rejected, abandoned, or in some way responsible for the situation.
- **Don't** say: "The pet went to sleep." Doing so may result in sleep problems by making the child fearful of meeting the same fate as his or her pet.
- **Don't** say: "The pet was sick and died" without immediately adding that being sick doesn't have to lead to dying. Otherwise, the child may become extremely fearful of illness.
- **Don't** stifle children's feelings by saying such things as: "Big boys and girls don't cry," or "It's only an animal. We'll get another one."
- **Do** allow the child to show and share feelings of anger, disappointment, and sadness, no matter how silly or irrational they may seem.

- **Do** be as positive a role model as possible, keeping in mind that children look to adults for direction and guidance.
- **Do** communicate to the child that you understand.
- **Do** let your child know that grief and mourning are normal.

Other books and videos on the subject of pet loss and bereavement are available from the American Animal Hospital Association; write or call AAHA, P.O. Box 150899, Denver, CO 80215-0899; (800) 252-2242.

From the Success File

A. Paul Bilger Jr., DVM, owner of the Walnut Hill Animal Hospital, in Dallas, Texas, says that he consistently gets more compliments and thank you's from clients for the thoughtful and helpful ways in which he and his staff deal with the death/euthanasia of pets than he does for any other single service he provides.

What came through when talking with Dr. Bilger was the genuine sensitivity and compassion he has for clients at such times. And that, I'm sure, explains his clients' gratitude.

I remember a small sticker that was placed on the office telephone of a Connecticut funeral home to remind employees of their important role. It read:

We have funerals every day.
The families we serve don't.

Help Lines

• Pet Loss Support Hotline, sponsored by the University of California, Davis. Call (916) 752-4200; 6:30 p.m. to 9:30 p.m., PST, Mon.-Fri.

• Grief counseling by Michigan State University veterinary student volunteers. Call (517) 432-2696; 6:30 p.m. to 9:30 p.m., EST, Tues., Wed., Thurs.

• Grief counseling by University of Florida-Gainesville veterinary student volunteers. Call (904) 338-2032; 7:00 p.m. to 9:00 p.m., EST, Mon.-Fri.

Exam-Room Etiquette

30

It's true that clients' reactions to your exam-room etiquette are often based more on *perception* than reality. Nonetheless, their impressions affect their satisfaction and, ultimately, their referrals. Here's a list of exam-room do's and don'ts based on client surveys we've done on the subject:

- **Don't** look at your watch. Doing so suggests you're either rushed or bored.
- **Do** call the client and pet by name. Otherwise, you'll appear cold and distant, or possibly, indifferent.
- **Do** refer to the pet by the proper gender. Pink and blue folders or stick-on labels are possible aids.
- **Don't** appear angry if the pet has an accident. Just say, "no problem," and clean it up yourself.
- **Don't** become indignant if the client wants to think things over or seek another opinion. It's his or her right.
- **Do** listen to clients with your eyes as well as your ears. Provide focused attention; for many clients, it's a priority.
- **Don't** criticize the judgment or skills of the client's previous veterinarian. Doing so insults the client's intelligence for having selected and trusted him or her.
- **Don't** leave the exam room without asking clients if they have any questions. Otherwise, they may forget to ask.
- **Don't** speak to the client while standing in the doorway, and especially not with your hand on the doorknob. Your body language shouts "No questions!"

The Secret of the
Philadelphia Hoagie

Reminiscing about his early life in Philadelphia, Joel Novack, a podiatric surgeon now practicing in Cleveland,
Ohio, recalled the sensational hoagies or "hero" sandwiches
made by a local chain of delicatessens. On one occasion, he
asked the proprietor what made their hoagies so much
better than those made by other delis.

"Is it the crusty bread?" Dr. Novack asked.

"No," the proprietor replied.

"Is it the special meats and cheeses?"

Again, the answer was "no."

"How about the olive oil? The condiments?"

"No," the proprietor said. "*It's everything.*"

"That simple lesson," Dr. Novack says, "made a lasting
impression. And years later, I realized the same principle
applies to practice. It's no one thing that leads to success.
It's everything."

In veterinary practice, this "total package" concept
means everything a client experiences when seeking veterinary services. It means:

- how clients and their pets are spoken to by staff members and doctors;
- how clients' concerns about their pets' symptoms or the
  cost of care are handled;
- how long clients are kept on "hold" when telephoning
  the hospital;

- whether clients see signs of competence and caring during their pet's examination or an assembly-line attitude;
- whether clients see a clean, well-maintained, odor-free, well-equipped hospital—or something less.

True differentiation in any endeavor seldom results from doing just one thing that much better than anyone else. It comes from doing *100 things just one percent better.*

3

Image Management

Moments of Truth

32

Jan Carlson, president and CEO of Scandinavian Airline Systems (SAS), is credited with popularizing the term "moment of truth." Taken from the lexicon of bull fighting, it refers to any episode in which a passenger (or prospective passenger) comes into contact with an SAS employee. For example, moments of truth include the points at which a passenger makes a reservation, checks in at the airport, boards the plane, retrieves luggage, or makes contact with an SAS employee during the flight.

As Carlson explains, "Nothing is more fragile than the fleeting contact between a customer in the marketplace and an employee on the front lines. When you establish contact, that's when you establish SAS."

In a recent year, SAS carried 10,000,000 passengers, each of whom experienced an average of five encounters with SAS employees. The result: 50,000,000 moments of truth to meet and if possible, exceed passengers' expectations for quality and service.

The moments of truth that occur in veterinary practice are equally important to your image and your clients' satisfaction. Consider the critical moments that occur when:

- a client or prospective client calls for an appointment
- a pet owner arrives at your practice
- a pet owner departs your practice
- a hospitalized animal is discharged
- the bill is presented

- there is an emergency
- the client is in the exam room.

In each case, the client's lasting impression is determined by how competent, concerned, accommodating, understanding, and professional you and your staff members are—not just on the first visit but *every time* a client calls or visits your practice.

Image Gap

33

When asked to guess the number of postgraduate courses their veterinarians have taken in the last six months, most clients say they haven't a clue. Such perceptions are disappointing—but not surprising, given the fact that most clients are never told about such courses. I call it an "image gap."

The *content* of the postgraduate courses you take is obviously out of most clients' realm, but merely *knowing that you've taken them* boosts clients' confidence in you. Builds their respect for your fees. Increases their loyalty to your practice. Don't lose these important benefits by keeping the continuing education that you, your associates, and your staff members take a secret.

An easy, low-key way to inform clients is to post a notice on a bulletin board in your reception area or mount it on a cardboard easel on the front counter. Suggested wording:

We will be away from the hospital from time to time in the coming year to attend postgraduate courses in veterinary medicine. Among them … (Here, list the dates, the individuals attending, the names of the courses, and short, nontechnical descriptions of what they're about.)

Posting such a message:

- makes clients aware of your and your staff's commitment to continuing education;
- alerts clients to your special interests and expertise (e.g., cardiology, orthopedics, herd health management);

- prompts inquiries about services that clients may not know you offer (e.g. feline medicine, nutrition, dentistry, behavioral counseling);
- explains your, your associate's, and your staff's extended absences from the hospital in a positive way.

Of course, not everyone will read such a notice or necessarily grasp its significance. But more than you might guess will read it—and be interested and impressed. If nothing else, it will help your practice avoid the image gap.

Another image gap: the one involving the disparity between the tremendous *investment* veterinarians make in their facilities and the amount clients typically *believe is invested.* What most clients overlook—and the reason they invariably *underestimate* the investment involved—is the *private ownership of your building and land.*

When made aware of these facts, clients are at first surprised; then *impressed*—as well they should be. The hospital and photographic tours described in this chapter help clients appreciate your investment and your commitment to patient care. And the following statement, perhaps included in your brochure or posted on a bulletin board, will help clients to better understand the whole picture:

Unlike the human hospital, these facilities are due entirely to private enterprise. Private funds are responsible for the construction and operation of the hospital. These funds represent a substantial investment in the community and in the protection of the community's public health and welfare.

51

Curb Appeal

34

In real estate jargon, "curb appeal" refers to the total impression a building creates from the street, including its overall condition, landscaping, and individual features. Even a practice with high visibility may have negative curb appeal—a dangerous combination that can discourage potential clients from entering.

Several factors work together to create the overall impression of your hospital, but this harmony can be destroyed by any of the following:

- a parking lot strewn with paper cups or windblown papers
- cracked pavement with overgrown weeds
- a sign in need of repair, repainting, or replacement
- poor outdoor lighting
- exterior paint that is peeling, blistered, stained, or faded
- masonry that needs to be repointed
- trees or shrubs in need of pruning, spraying, or replacement
- windows with cracked or dirty panes
- a roof with missing shingles
- wilted plants or flowers
- an unsightly doorway.

It's all too easy to grow accustomed to the small flaws that diminish your hospital's curb appeal. To keep your standards high, ask three or four of your best clients to evaluate your facility's exterior as if they were seeing it for the first time. You might ask them, for example, "Have we overlooked any problems?" or "If you had $1,000 to spend, what would you do to improve the hospital's curb appeal?" By seeking a fresh perspective, you'll be more attuned to the wishes of your regular clients and more apt to coax prospective clients inside.

35

People Judge the Unknown by the Known

Tip

It's not whether you're worth what you charge; it's whether the public thinks you're worth what you charge. For many people, one of the determining factors in such a judgment is how you're dressed. Ask yourself: Does what you and your staff wear when seeing clients project the right image for your practice? Is it in keeping with your level of expertise and your fee structure?

In answer to the question: "What is the best change you've ever made in your practice?" Bob Paulsen, DVM, told me: "It was the day I put on a necktie to make a farm call. What happened," he went on to say, "was an immediate change in the attitude of producers and of farm and feed-lot personnel. And it set the stage for charging for what I *know* rather than what I *do* on such calls."

Roger M. Meads, DVM, a prominent dairy practitioner and consultant concurs: "You may have good ideas," he says, "but clients won't take you seriously if you aren't properly dressed."

"We have nine veterinarians in our practice," Dr. Meads says, "and we are never seen without a necktie. If the hour is 9 a.m. or 9 p.m., midnight or 5 a.m., and whether we're pulling a calf, treating milk fever, or providing any other veterinary service, our DVMs always wear a necktie."

"We find it easier," he adds, "to charge professional fees if we *look professional*."

But this Success Secret isn't really about neckties. It's about *image* and the impact it has on your credibility and fee structure. I've met practitioners who insist on comfortable clothing—who "do their own thing" and let their staffs do the same. I think they're making a big mistake by ignoring a reality of the marketplace: the tendency of people to judge the *unknown* by the *known.*

Is Your Practice
Sending Mixed Messages?

36

A veterinary practice that prides itself on clinical excellence yet allows a serious odor problem to go unchecked sends mixed messages to clients and raises a legitimate question: Is the quality of care provided to patients as poor as the hospital maintenance?

Veterinarians and staff members in such a practice are often desensitized to the smell—and therefore unaware of the problem. Clients, of course, are aware of the problem but seldom complain about it. Sales reps are reluctant to mention the problem as well. So the odor problems persist, undermining the hospital's image and credibility—and possibly driving clients away.

We all know the importance of proper ventilation, air-purification systems, disinfectants, and materials for the walls, ceilings, and floors that don't absorb odors and moisture. Equally important, however, is a *commitment,* starting at the top with the practice owner, to create an odor-free veterinary hospital.

An American Airlines brochure entitled, "Now More Than Ever *Cleanliness* Makes The Difference Between Airlines" illustrates the point: "Cost cutting will never come before cleanliness at American Airlines. Keeping our planes clean is a reflection of an attitude that runs through our entire organization. American is committed to doing the job right. Not just sometimes. But all the time."

Continued

Cleanliness also makes a difference—some might say an important difference—between practices. The question: Is it a commitment you and your staff want to make?

Reality Check

Does your hospital have an odor problem? If your clients never compliment you on how clean and odor-free your hospital is, chances are your hospital does *have a problem.*

Is Your Busy Practice Sending the Wrong Message?

"Nothing succeeds like success" goes the old saying. And looking busy does say you're successful. In fact, it's a great image. Good for business. But if your "busy-ness" looks excessive, it can send the wrong message, antagonizing clients and discouraging referrals.

An example of such overkill: veterinarians who complain (perhaps brag) how overworked, understaffed, rushed, and behind schedule they are. They go on about the long hours, nighttime emergencies, and weekends with which they must contend. Or they always appear breathless and time-pressured. All of that may be true, but it's the wrong message to send to clients who are paying for your time and expertise and expect someone who is alert, attentive, and at his or her best.

Solution: If your practice is truly that busy, hire an associate or additional full- or part-time employees to shoulder some of the work. Or delegate some of what you do to others, including emergency clinics. Most important, when telling clients or prospective clients how busy your practice is, stop short of making it sound as if you are too busy to see new clients or to give existing clients the time and attention they deserve.

Food for Thought

Would an accountant who appears overworked, understaffed, rushed, and behind schedule at tax time give you confidence your tax return will be given his or her closest scrutiny and judgment?

38

The Problem No One Mentions but Everyone Notices

The problem to which I'm referring isn't bad breath. But it's close. It's *badly neglected teeth* that have conspicuous stains on them or that are noticeably chipped, missing, or have large spaces between them. The problem isn't so much the cosmetic effect; it's what it "says" about your personal hygiene (or lack thereof). In some people's minds, such *perceived neglect* could raise doubts about your judgment and credibility as a healthcare provider.

The good news is that in most cases such dental defects are easily corrected through these techniques:

- Bleaching (tooth whitening) is a procedure best done by the dentist or with a prescribed at-home system.
- Bonding is the application of newly developed composite resins to the teeth. The technique not only covers stains completely but also rebuilds chipped or cracked teeth, closes gaps, and builds up old, eroded teeth to make them younger looking.
- With laminate veneers, a thin layer of acrylic or porcelain is bonded to the outer surface of the tooth to improve its appearance. The results can be spectacular.

Take time today for a no-excuse smile analysis and, if needed, see a dentist.

Pet Therapy

Want to do a kindness for others that will have a positive impact on your practice as well? Consider participating in a "pet-visitation program" at a local nursing home or healthcare facility.

Gene Rinderknecht, DVM, started such a program in Newton, Iowa. Once a week, he and his staff members take well-socialized pets to a nursing home for the residents to hold, pet, and talk to. The residents enjoy reminiscing about their own pets, and the attendants marvel that the visits coax some seniors to smile or talk for the first time in months.

From the start, the residents have eagerly anticipated "Visitation Day." Their spirits improve, and the event often brings a liveliness and communication between them that continues long after the visits. "Brightening the lives of some very dear folks was one of the most gratifying things I've ever done," Dr. Rinderknecht says.

If you'd like more information about starting such a program, contact the AVMA, (800) 248-2862; the Delta Society, (206) 226-7357; or the Center to Study Human-Animal Relationships and Environments, (612) 625-5741.

40

Babies and Pets

Looking for innovative community-service projects? James Bacon, DVM, of Somerset, N.J., found a receptive audience to "Babies and Pets," a 30-minute lecture he gave to 50 parents and parents-to-be at Robert Wood Johnson University Hospital in New Brunswick, N.J. Dr. Bacon's program provided guidelines for parents bringing home a new pet and for pet owners bringing home a new baby.

Among the subjects he covered: how to introduce babies and pets to each other; how to deal with the jealousy and rivalry that pets and babies often show in such situations; and how to avoid such transmissible health problems as Lyme disease, toxoplasmosis, and internal and external parasites. Dr. Bacon also provided handouts, including the booklet, "Introducing Your Dog to Your New Baby" (available from Quaker Oats Professional Services, 585 Hawthorne Ct., Galesburg, IL 61401).

Will such community-service projects generate new clients for your practice? Perhaps. But don't let that be your prime intent. As Dr. Bacon says, "What goes around, comes around."

The Child/Companion Animal Bond

Recognizing a need for an educational, hands-on program to help young children properly care for their pets, prevent animal bites, and perhaps overcome a fear of companion animals, Mona L. Gitter, DVM, of Noblesville, Ind., developed a two-hour program entitled "Kids and Pets."

With the help of a staff member, some friendly dogs, cats, and baby cockatiels (always a big hit with the children), and sometimes a stuffed toy dog, the class is periodically offered at her Noblesville Square Animal Clinic at a cost of $12 per child with all proceeds going to the Indianapolis Humane Society.

To publicize the class, Dr. Gitter includes an announcement in her practice newsletter and circulates a notice to the local pediatricians, pediatric dentist, OB/GYNs, pharmacists, and library. Among the participants in a recent class: a child who played too roughly with the family's puppy and another who was terrified of dogs. In both cases, Dr. Gitter's instruction proved helpful—to the delight of the children and especially their parents.

Dr. Gitter, who lectures frequently at local schools, recommends such classes be limited to 10 children within a narrow age group (for example, five to eight years) to simplify the instruction and avoid intimidation of younger participants by older children.

Such a program offers numerous benefits: It fosters the child/companion animal bond, teaches responsible pet ownership, develops client loyalty, and in the big picture, is good for the image of your practice.

Helpful Resource

The Auxiliary to the AVMA offers a unique collection of three educational animal care videos entitled "Petpourri." Each is designed for a specific grade level: K-1st grade; 2nd-4th grade; and 5th-7th grade. The K-1 program costs $7; the other two cost $10 each.

The programs are four to eight minutes long, and they utilize animation to explain the care and needs of pets. To order, contact: AVMA Auxiliary, 1931 N. Meacham Road, Schaumburg, IL 60173-4360; (708) 397-6651.

4

Front-Desk Service

First Impressions

42

First scenario: A client calls your practice, identifies herself, and requests an appointment. The receptionist, not recognizing the name, asks the caller: "Are you a client here?"

That seemingly innocuous question can have an extremely negative impact—especially on a client who's been to the hospital on numerous occasions, spent substantial dollars along the way, and made several referrals to your practice.

Unfortunately, clients rarely complain about such matters. But their good feelings about your practice and personnel may be diminished.

The problem is easily solved: If your receptionist is in doubt whether a caller is an established client, suggest she simply ask: "When did you last see the doctor?"

Second scenario: A new client calls to schedule a first appointment. Consider asking your receptionist to say, "If you have any questions to ask the doctor, may I suggest you write them down on a piece of paper and bring the list with you. We'll make sure all of your questions are answered."

This simple gesture makes the client's first call to your practice a memorable moment of truth (see Success Secret 32). It also signals a sincere interest in the client's needs and differentiates your practice from others.

How to Activate "Inactive" Clients

43

Of all the ways to generate revenue, none is more logical (or easier) than getting clients who haven't been to the practice in one or two years to return with their pets for needed veterinary services.

As a start, ask your receptionist to call 25 randomly selected inactive clients, and explain:

In reviewing our records, I see that Snoopy hasn't had booster vaccinations (or heartworm or fecal tests, dental cleaning, or whatever is indicated on the chart) since (date). I'm just calling to see if you would like to make an appointment at this time.

Your receptionist may learn that (a) the client has moved away; (b) the pet has died; or (c) the client is now using another veterinarian. Or she may hear that "Snoopy's doing fine and doesn't need an appointment."

But let's focus on the easy-to-activate clients who say: (a) "Has it really been that long?" (b) "I know it's been a long time. I've been meaning to call you;" or (c) "I've been waiting for you to call me." Needless to say, only a handful of such responses will more than warrant telephoning the balance of your inactive clients.

A few suggestions:

• If your receptionist isn't comfortable making such calls,

Reality Check

If you haven't discussed the importance of booster vaccinations, heartworm and fecal tests, and so on with clients during hospital visits, it's unlikely telephone calls will do the job. Also, attempts to get clients to make appointments by using fear as a motivator and stressing the consequences of further delay may be construed as high pressure and resented.

ask someone else to do it. A willing caller will be more believable to your clients.

- If clients can't be reached during hospital hours, consider paying one of your staff members to make such calls from home in the evening and reimburse him or her for telephone usage.

- Most important: Remind the person making the calls to keep them *low-key*. They're not meant to be "sales calls"; they're just a reminder. For example, if the client says, "It's not a good time to talk," don't persist, saying, "this will take just a minute." Instead, offer to call the client at another, more convenient time.

The fact is: Many clients *want* to do what's best for their pets—but become busy or forgetful. These clients in particular will appreciate such a call—and proceed to make an appointment.

Telephone Shoppers = Golden Opportunity

44

How many telephone shoppers call your practice every day? If you don't know or simply consider such calls a nuisance, consider these findings: My company's research indicates that only *some* of these telephone shoppers are looking for the *lowest* cost; others are calling for a variety of reasons and, if handled properly, may become clients— excellent clients in some cases.

Here's a proven protocol for converting more telephone shoppers into clients:

1. Don't hesitate to quote a fee for the procedure in question, or, if more appropriate, a *range* of fees. Refusal to do so may strike some callers as unreasonable—if not suspicious.

Tip: Ask callers if they're shopping and if so, suggest that they make sure the fees quoted elsewhere are "all inclusive" (as yours are). Doing so will eliminate the confusion created by "low-ball" quotes from other practices.

2. Offer to send telephone shoppers a hospital brochure with information about your training, scope of practice, and hospital facilities.

Tip: If the call is about an ovariohysterectomy, end the conversation by saying: "Remember, this is a once-in-a-lifetime procedure for your pet. Wherever you choose to have it done, make sure it's done right."

3. Call a few days later to ask if the client received the brochure and if he or she has any questions or would like to make an appointment. If the person is undecided, con-

sider offering a brief, no-charge visit to meet the doctor and see your facility.

Obtaining only a few new clients you may have previously missed will more than justify the time and expense involved.

From The Success Files

Clients inquiring about the cost of a spay or vaccinations can be sent a narrative explaining exactly what's involved in far greater detail than would be practical to give over the telephone.

Patricia Kennedy, DVM, hospital director of the eight-doctor Jefferson Animal Hospital and Emergency Center in Louisville, Ky., provides a one-page sheet she wrote entitled: "Spaying Your Pet At Jefferson Animal Hospital." The sheet describes the diagnostic and medical workups required before the procedure; the surgery itself; the many safety measures taken along the way; and the strict recovery standards following surgery. It's impressive—and helps clients realize that a spay is, in fact, major abdominal surgery. The written information also gives "telephone shoppers" something other than cost to think about.

Indecisive Clients

45

Do your clients ever ask your staff members if your recommendations, such as a pre-surgical blood screen, are really necessary? If so, how does your staff respond? If they answer, "no," the problem is obvious. But if your employees immediately affirm the recommendation, you may still have a problem.

Why? Because clients may interpret this "yes" as a self-serving and economically motivated response rather than a careful consideration of the pet's best interest. In fact, if clients later feel they were talked into something that wasn't really necessary, they may develop "buyer's remorse" and refuse to pay the bill.

Chris Lembke, the office manager of the Animal Medical Center in Brandon, Fla., recommends that rather than immediately answering the client's question, the staff member say, "What makes you ask?" Most of the time, she notes, clients express an underlying fear or need more information. By asking the client about his or her concerns, you can better address the specific problem.

The point, Lembke says, is to keep clients involved in the decision-making process rather than dictating your recommendations in a heavy-handed way. "Our clients much prefer this helpful, low-key approach," she says.

How to Handle Complaints

46

Disgruntled clients can complain about countless things: a long wait to see the doctor; higher than expected fees; a pet that's sent home dirty and smelly. As they say, it comes with the territory. But how such complaints are handled can be critical to client retention. The following ground rules may be helpful for your front-desk personnel, to whom the complaints are invariably directed:

- Always assume clients have a legitimate complaint. Even if they don't, they think they do—so hear them out, and don't interrupt. When clients tell you what's bothering them, show concern. If appropriate, take notes. Such actions show you're interested and paying attention. If a client has overreacted to the situation or exaggerated the complaint, he or she will become calmer simply by seeing that you are sympathetic and responsive.
- Concede before you contend. Agree with what the client says before responding. For example, *I can understand why you are upset. I'd feel the same way if I were in your shoes.* Realizing you're not defensive or argumentative about the situation, clients will tend to be more reasonable and receptive to what you have to say. In fact, a little sympathetic understanding at this point can quickly turn a "lemon" into lemonade.
- Whenever possible, do what you can do to resolve the situation in the client's favor. Admit your mistake. Apologize. Offer a free bath for the pet or a complimen-

tary bottle of vitamins or whatever is appropriate. If that falls short, ask the client, "what can we do to make you happy?" And be prepared to do it. In the long run, it will be worth it.

Management expert Tom Peters says that a well-handled complaint usually breeds more loyalty than existed before the incident occurred.

For Staff's Eyes Only

A sign in the staff lounge of a Midwest practice reads: "Never let a client go away mad without first seeing the doctor—unless it was the doctor who made the client mad."

Parting Questions

47

A pet is being discharged following hospitalization. Consider telling the owner: "This is what we fed Pepper while he was in the hospital—and he really liked it. Would you like to take a bag home?"

Another scenario: The hospital visit is over. The client is at the front desk, making payment. The receptionist, with the client/patient records before her, has a perfect opportunity to ask: "Do you have enough heartworm medication (or pet food or flea-control supplies or whatever the records indicate are being used)?" An even lower-key question: "Is there anything else you need while you're here?"

In both of the above scenarios, you may be surprised how many clients will thank you for the recommendation or for reminding them—and then purchase something.

From the Success File

On farm calls, David Farst, DVM, of Arcanum, Ohio, uses both types of parting questions—usually as he's about to leave: "Do you have enough mastitis tubes (or penicillin salve or calf scours pills, or, as above, whatever the records indicate is being used)?" he asks. Or he'll just ask, "Is there anything else you need while I'm here?"

"About 75 percent of the time," Dr. Farst says, "clients remember something (or an additional service) they need— or sometimes, they have a question that when answered leads to additional work."

Useful References

- *The Veterinary Receptionist's Handbook* by M.T. McClister, DVM, and Amy Midgley (Veterinary Medicine Publishing Group, 1996) includes such topics as making a good first impression; answering commonly asked questions; the importance of diagnostic tests and parasite control; common medical problems; and handling emergencies. Call (800) 255-6864.
- The American Animal Hospital Association (AAHA) offers training publications and videotapes on such topics as basic telephone techniques; time management; collections; and how to handle dissatisfied clients and emergency situations. Call (800) 252-2242 or (303) 986-2800.
- The American Veterinary Medical Association (AVMA) offers training publications including "Telephone Courtesy and Client Service"; "Beyond Customer Service—Keeping Clients For Life"; and "Client Satisfaction—The Other Half of Your Job." Call (708) 925-8070.
- Hill's Pet Nutrition, Inc. offers "Hill's Health Care Connection," a self-study course in clinical nutrition and practice development for all members of a veterinary health care team. Call (800) 255-0499.

Notes

5

Client
Education

Do Your Clients See
the Whole Picture?

48

Looking at the picture below, what do you see?

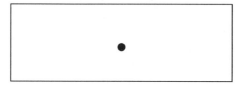

Seminar audiences typically report seeing "a black dot." What they're missing, of course, is the much larger, more significant *rectangle* in which the dot appears.

In making judgments, people often see only the obvious or what appears obvious from their perspective. And in doing so, they overlook the significant. In the same way, clients often focus on fees, and in the process, overlook the clinical and economic significance of such important factors as:

- a fully equipped, state-of-the-art veterinary hospital
- the many steps involved before, during, and after a surgical procedure
- the utilization of such support services as radiology, endoscopy, ultrasonography, intensive care, anesthesiology, pathology, nursing care, and pharmacy.

Clients who overlook such significant factors are unable to appreciate the quality of care or the behind-the-scene services provided at your hospital. Some may decide they were overcharged; others may begin to look for lower-cost alternatives.

Client education is the answer. Lots of it. That's why so many of the following "secrets" pertain to helping clients see the "whole picture."

Seeing the Whole Picture in Food Animal Practice

Some dairy producers still believe that herd-health management is an unnecessary expense. But the fact is: The return on investment for mastitis control is extremely high in terms of improved milk production, lower labor costs, lower veterinary bills, decreased need for drugs, less discarded milk, and fewer animals lost to death and premature culling.

To help clients see the "whole picture," client education is the answer.

Annual Geriatric Exams

49

One reason many clients don't make appointments for annual examinations for their geriatric dogs is that they don't realize that dogs age faster than humans. In many cases, they've never been told—at least not in meaningful and memorable terms.

The table below is adapted from a handout used by W.H. Crago, DVM, of Youngstown, Ohio, to explain how old a dog is in human years. It helps make the point that an annual physical examination is just as important for a dog approaching middle age as it is for a middle-aged owner.

Dog's age	Human's age
6 months	10 years
12 months	15 years
2 years	24 years
4 years	32 years
6 years	40 years
8 years	48 years
10 years	56 years
12 years	64 years
14 years	72 years
16 years	80 years
18 years	88 years
20 years	96 years

Another highly effective way to communicate the fact that pets age faster than humans is to say:

The calendar year represents about 1.5 percent of an average American's life span of 75 years. But the same 12 months represents 5 to 10 percent of a dog or cat's 10- to 20-year life span. An animal's organs aren't genetically programmed to last as long as those of humans, so health problems often manifest themselves faster.

In other words, a client who waits two years to bring in a 10-year-old cat may have watched 10 to 20 percent of the animal's life pass by without veterinary care—at a time when the patient needs it most. That's comparable to a 70-year-old man or woman not seeing a physician for seven to 14 years.

This message, adapted from *Practice Health: Ways To Enhance Your Cash Flow* (Hill's Pet Nutrition, Inc., 1993), is one of the most important you and your staff can convey to clients when discussing the health benefits of nutrition and preventive care. It's also a sound reason to implement geriatric protocols for your patients.

To clients who comply, say, "I wish all pet owners were as conscientious as you are. Their pets would be a lot healthier." It's true. It's a well-deserved compliment, and it has reinforcement value.

50

Must Reading for Veterinarians

The November 1994 issue of *Prevention* magazine, which reaches 3 million readers, includes the article "Anesthesia for Animals" by Dr. Amy Marder of Tufts University School of Veterinary Medicine. It's a must-read for all veterinarians.

In the article, Dr. Marder discusses the importance of a pre-anesthetic exam and subsequent lab tests, especially for older pets. Dr. Marder advises pet owners to ask these questions before they give the go-ahead for anesthesia:

- What is the risk of anesthesia for my pet?
- What type of anesthesia will be used and how will it be tailored to my pet's needs?
- Will an endotracheal tube (which the article explains) be inserted into my pet?
- Will someone assist in the procedure...and monitor my pet through recovery?
- Does the veterinarian have a "crash cart" for emergencies?

Answer such questions carefully. A response clients perceive to be evasive, confusing, or patronizing is counterproductive, while a true educational effort is likely to make clients more appreciative of such precautions—and more accepting of your fees.

If you'd like copies of the article to distribute, contact Carol Spiciarich; her address: *Prevention*, 33 E. Minor Street, Emmaus, PA 18098-0099; fax: (610) 967-7654.

Photographic Hospital Tour

51

It's truly unfortunate that few if any clients ever see more of the veterinary hospitals they visit than the reception area and exam rooms. That limited exposure leads them to vastly underestimate the wide range of hospital services available and the expertise, equipment, and investment required to provide such services. Unfortunately, this limited view leads some clients to resent the costs of hospitalization, surgery, anesthesiology, and the like, or worse, feel they were overcharged.

One solution is a hospital tour—but that can be time-consuming and impractical. An alternative is a *photographic* tour, which can be accomplished with either a photo album or framed photographs in the reception area. People like to look at pictures, especially those with people they know and those with pets.

Consider hiring a professional photographer to take color photographs of your surgery room (with you capped, gowned, masked, gloved and perhaps working with a surgical assistant); and of the pathology lab, with a technician at work and surrounded by diagnostic equipment. You also might include a series of photographs depicting diagnostic imaging, anesthesiology, dentistry, nursing care, emergency services, the pharmacy, and so on.

You can add human interest by including photographs of all of your associates and staff members working, or perhaps just holding a variety of companion animals. Most important is to include captions that indicate the name of the individual, an explanation of what he or she is doing, and the important role the job plays in quality care and hospital safety. Photographs of such important support services as medical records, housekeeping and maintenance, and even your library can add interest as well.

Note: The American Animal Hospital Association (AAHA) offers its members an attractive binder entitled "Behind The Scenes," which contains 22 laminated pages; 3 1/2" x 5" stock photographs of the above-mentioned services (which can be covered by your own), and pre-printed captions that explain the importance and meaning of AAHA standards. The price is $29.95. Call AAHA: (303) 986-2800 or (800) 252-2242.

If a photographic tour of your hospital makes even a few clients realize "it's just like a real hospital," it will be well worth the effort and expense.

The Most Impressive Part of Your Hospital

52

"The operating room of most veterinary hospitals is one of the most important, impressive, and costliest areas of the facility," says Fred J. Born, DVM, Fond du Lac, Wis. "Unfortunately," he adds, "most clients don't get to see it."

That's why Dr. Born installed a 6' x 4' window in the operating room of the Town and Country Veterinary Clinic. The window allows clients to see the operating room from the hallway. In selected cases, clients view an actual surgery, although not usually on their own pets.

When clients bring their pets in for a pre-surgical exam, they're asked if they would "like to take a peek at the operating room." "Many express an interest," Dr. Born says. "What they see is a spotlessly clean, fully equipped OR. If a surgery is in progress, they see the surgeon (capped, gowned, masked, and gloved) and sometimes a surgical assistant. What they don't see—thanks to surgical drapes and table height—is the patient or the incision site.

"A minute at the viewing window immediately raises clients' 'Veterinary IQ,' and lets them appreciate our facilities, skills, and hospital protocol. And you frequently hear such comments as 'it's just like a real hospital' or 'just like human surgery.' That insight alone is well worth the time it takes to escort clients to the viewing window. What's nice, too, is that you seldom hear complaints about fees."

Consider giving your clients a peek at the most impressive part of your hospital.

I.T.A.E.Y.W.L.T.A.M.?

53

I recently interviewed a physician who'd posted the above letters on the back of his exam room door. "The letters," he said, "are to remind me to ask every patient before leaving the room, *Is there anything else you would like to ask me?*"

"Great idea," I said. "But doesn't that open the door for some questions that might be rather time-consuming to answer?"

"Surprisingly, not very often," he said. "Most times, it's a question the patient meant to ask but forgot, and it's easily answered. When it is a question that requires a lengthy answer, I either give the patient literature that has the necessary information, ask a qualified staff person to answer the question, or set up another appointment to discuss the matter more in-depth."

You, too, can benefit from I.T.A.E.Y.W.L.T.A.M. The extra time it takes is worth it, and your clients will appreciate the extra service, care, and attention. I.T.A.E.Y.W.L.T.A.M. also differentiates you from high-volume/assembly-line offices in which practitioners can't or won't answer clients' questions.

6

Personnel Management and Motivation

The Magic Power of Appreciation

54

Psychologist William James wrote, "The deepest principle in human nature is the craving to be appreciated." Notice that he didn't say "wish" or "desire" or even "longing." He said *craving*.

Finding something nice to say about others may seem trivial, but it satisfies a universal hunger. Unfortunately, however, people who feel appreciation often fail to express it. They become inhibited, forgetful, busy with their day-to-day priorities.

Some people mistakenly assume that other people's need for appreciation can be internally met—"she knows she does a good job." Even if that were true, a verbal pat on the back or a written note of thanks for "a job well done" provides the kind of psychological satisfaction for which there is no substitute. (When President Reagan wrote "Very Good" on the draft of a speech prepared by speech writer Peggy Noonan, she cut the words out, taped them to her blouse, and wore them all day).

The list of candidates for appreciation is endless if you stop and think of the many people who contribute to the success of your practice. For a start, thank your staff for their efforts and dedication and for making your hospital look good. I guarantee it'll make their day! And by expressing appreciation, you may start a chain reaction. Praise begets praise. People will like you more for saying kind things, and you will feel good for having said them.

Reality Check

In the course of conducting seminars for a wide range of professional groups, I've asked more than 1,000 doctors to consider the following statement: "I let my employees know when they're doing a good job" and then rate themselves on a scale of 1 to 5 (1=never; 5=always). The average response: 4.4. So far, so good.

At these same seminars, I've also asked staff members to consider the statement: "The doctor lets me know when I'm doing a good job," using the same rating scale. The average response: 1.7.

The difference between the amount of positive feedback doctors say they give employees and the amount employees say they get is what I call the Feedback Gap. And often it's the underlying cause of employee resentment, diminished productivity, and turnover.

Tip

One clue to a job applicant's need for appreciation is his or her answer to the question: In your last job, did you receive the recognition and appreciation you felt you deserved?

A Flexible Sick-Leave Policy

55

Tip

An Alaska practitioner credits two hours of vacation time for employees who don't use sick leave during an entire calendar month. A staff member not taking sick leave for six months receives an extra day and a half.

Additional Tip

You can get a sense of an applicant's attitude toward sick days by asking: What constitutes a good attendance record? What are good reasons for missing work?

What happens when employees are needed at home to care for a sick child, spouse, or other family member? Do they call in "sick" and take the day off? Do they come to work—yet remain distracted by the at-home situation? The answer depends on several factors, one of which is the flexibility of your sick-leave policy.

An employee benefit that is becoming more widely offered extends conventional sick leave to include other times when family members are ill. Called "family sick leave," it eliminates the need to fake an illness and then lie about it. And in the end, it doesn't cost you any more.

Typically, family sick leave is computed at the rate of one-half day for each month worked (after a 90-day probationary period), up to a total of six days a year. What about unused sick days? Increasingly, employees are being paid for them. Doing so provides an incentive to get to work for those undecided about making the effort.

An alternative way of dealing with unused sick days is to accumulate them in a "paid leave bank," up to a maximum of 20 to 30 days per employee. These days can then be used for such emergencies as a major illness or surgery, allowing employees to take the time needed for recuperation without losing pay.

Keep in mind that flexible personnel policies are helpful in attracting and retaining top-notch employees.

Are You A
Do-It-Yourself DVM?

Many veterinarians are performing tasks in their practices that could be done just as well, perhaps better, and definitely at less cost, by *non-veterinarians*. The tasks fall in all areas of the practice; some are related to management, some to medicine, some are just routine chores.

Many veterinarians justify their failure to delegate by saying: "If I want it done right, I have to do it myself;" or "It's easier (or faster) to do it myself." Unfortunately, this line of reasoning becomes a self-fulfilling prophecy. Employees can't learn to do what veterinarians insist on doing themselves. So the doctors keep on doing what they've always done.

If you are a do-it-yourself DVM, there is a lot to be gained if you are willing to loosen the reins a little and to allow qualified employees to tackle new assignments and take on more responsibility. Delegation frees you to do more of the things only you can do: see more clients and patients, do more thorough exams, provide quality care, do more surgery, spend more time with clients. You'll be less rushed, have more free time, and be less stressed.

Employees interested in personal growth, job enrichment, and broader responsibilities will benefit as well. Their earnings potential will increase, as will their interest, pride, and satisfaction in their work.

Tip

Consider the impact of saving only 20 minutes a day through delegation. That would add up to two hours a week—or the equivalent of two weeks of practice a year!

57

Incentive Plans: Weighing the Risks

Before you implement an incentive program for your employees, consider these potential drawbacks, all from veterinarians who've tried such plans:

- In some cases, employees become over-eager and high-pressure clients into buying elective procedures or over-the-counter products. Some clients resent it; others who say yes later experience "buyer's remorse."
- Some clients learn of the incentive program—perhaps from a former, disgruntled employee—and begin to fear that the *bonus*, not the pet's well-being, is behind your employees' recommendations.
- When incentive pay is distributed equally among full-time employees, team spirit can quickly deteriorate if one staff member believes he or she works harder and thus deserves more income than the others.
- Employees can become dependent on incentive pay—and reluctant to relinquish it—especially when they aren't responsible for a business slow-down.

Give incentive plans careful consideration. In our surveys, we've found that while they may sound good on paper, and may work well in the short run, they can create more problems than they solve.

Group Pride

Dr. Rensis Likert of the University of Michigan says that high-performance organizations are invariably characterized by feelings of "group pride." His studies indicate that a decisive factor in such cases is the degree to which people:

- meet and interact with each other
- identify with one another
- seek to achieve organizational goals through collaborative efforts.

The football teams that win the Super Bowl meet each of those requirements. So do high-performance veterinary practices. And you *sense* it the moment you walk in the door. Staff members speak of "*our* hospital, *our* practice, *our* clients" with such obvious pride, joy, and enthusiasm that you *know* they have their hearts in their work.

Such pride and team spirit starts at the top—with you— and even the simplest gesture can make a difference. For example, introducing an animal handler who's assisting you in the exam room to the client—perhaps adding, "Linda's the best; we're lucky to have her"—sends a very different message than failing to acknowledge her.

From the Success File

To express pride in his professional "family" and enable clients to relate to his hospital's 25 staff members on a personal level, John M. Todd, DVM, founder of the Manassas

Animal Hospital in Manassas, Va., assembled a leather-bound photo album with color, on-the-job photos of each staff member. The album, which is kept in the reception area, also includes a short write-up on each person. A sample entry reads:

Sharon Crawford, Receptionist. Sharon says her life-long love of animals brought her to work for Manassas Animal Hospital. She has computer experience, which has proved extremely valuable in her receptionist duties. Sharon is also involved with extensive volunteer work, including the SPCA and nursing-home visitations with companion animals.

Staff members appreciate the recognition and respect conveyed by the album. And clients enjoy the opportunity to learn more about the healthcare givers who attend so capably to them and their pets.

Lively Staff Meetings

59

Staff meetings exemplify the kind of activities associated with high-performance organizations and are a proven way to foster group pride. But to be effective, staff meetings need to be *interactive*.

If your staff meetings have become a waste of time—if the participants sit in stony silence with their arms folded, contributing little if anything to the discussion and waiting for the meeting to end—give the following tested tips a try. They may revive the meetings by making them livelier, more interactive, more productive, and more fun.

- Ask your staff what they consider the best time for a meeting and pay them if it's not during regular office hours. (Asking them to stay late or come in early is starting a staff meeting on the wrong foot and dooming it to certain failure.) If lunch time is selected, make it your treat. You'll see the difference this one change will make in people's attitude.
- Give advance notice of both the date and agenda of staff meetings. Encourage staff members to add appropriate topics of their own.
- Rotate the leadership of the meeting among doctors, associates, technicians, the hospital manager, and all staff members—on a volunteer basis. Make it an *opportunity*, not an *obligation*.
- Stick to the agenda. If a real give-and-take discussion is the goal, the meeting leader should make short state-

Reality Check

Carefully consider whether to schedule a staff meeting on "hospital time" or "staff time." These two options send two very different messages about the importance of the meeting and the value of each person's input.

ments not speeches. Pass over minor points. Encourage participation. Be ready to listen. At the staff meetings held by Jan Wolf, DVM, of Kenosha, Wisc., participants use "clickers" to signal someone who is being unnecessarily negative, long-winded, or otherwise out of order. It keeps the discussion positive and on-target.

- Whenever possible, implement changes in hospital policies and procedures by consensus. People tend to be more supportive of changes that they have a say in making than of decisions made unilaterally by the boss and passed down to them.
- Schedule staff meetings as often as they are needed and as long as they continue to be productive.

To start off the meeting, consider asking: In what ways can we improve the:

- hospital decor
- appointment scheduling
- collections
- reminder system?

Or you might ask: In what ways can we save:

- time
- money
- needed hospital space?

Promoting A
Culture of Change

60

As you have undoubtedly surmised, creating a high-performance practice is not a set formula—it's a "mind set." And that mind set must lead to constant action and constant innovation. While these actions may at first seem deliberate and awkward, they eventually will become a way of life in your practice.

Ask yourself: Do you embrace change? Do your staff members know you desire on-going improvements? Is this something you think about—and communicate to them?

If change is overdue in your practice, consider holding what Gene M. Kangley, DDS, and his staff in Pompano Beach, Fla., call a "How We Can Do It Better" meeting.

First, Dr. Kangley asks everyone in the office to submit a list of practice-related matters that need change and/or improvement. Two weeks before the meeting, a compiled list is circulated. I saw one list with 13 items, among them: security measures needed in the office and general building area; remodeling of the bathroom; medical emergency procedures; protocol for a new patient emergency visit; out-of-office public relations; and appointment scheduling.

The meetings are held quarterly on a Friday from noon to 2:00 p.m. with a catered lunch. Follow-up meetings are held each Monday from 8:30 to 9:00 a.m. to monitor the progress of the agreed-upon changes and to review the week's schedule. It's a team approach to making *change* an ongoing process.

Role Playing

61

How would your receptionist reply to a client who, when told the charges for his or her hospital visit, replies, "I forgot my checkbook." or "Whew! That's expensive."? What is the best way to deal with such situations? Would other staff members handle them differently?

Role playing may help answer these questions. It's a training activity, typically used during staff meetings, to help people improve their communication skills. Here's how it works: The staff meeting leader (doctor, hospital manager, or staff member) recruits two volunteers to play the roles of receptionist and client. The two then act out a problematic situation, improvising as they go, while the rest of the group observes. Later, everyone critiques what was said and brainstorms for improvement.

Your staff can role play any number of scenarios—for example, interactions with a telephone shopper, a disgruntled client, or a mischievous child. And they can assume either role in any given situation. The objective? To sensitize everyone to the diplomacy needed in difficult situations, to agree on the best response, and to practice saying it in a non-threatening environment.

A few ground rules: Make critiques impersonal by using fictitious names for every character or by simply referring to them as "the client" and "the staff member." After the role play, ask the person playing the client how he or she felt about the staff member's response. Also ask the group how they might have handled the situation differently. Vote on the best ways to respond in these situations, and then use them as models for similar future encounters.

Done properly, role playing can be a lot of fun—and a great learning experience. Consider these starter ideas:

- A client picks up a pet following hospitalization and hits the ceiling when she finds the pet dirty and smelly.
- A client becomes grief-stricken over the death of a beloved pet.
- A client, tearful as her dog is admitted for boarding, says, "He's never been away from me overnight before."
- When asked for payment, the client says: "I'm all out of checks" or "Can I pay you on Friday?"

Comparative Comprehension Rates

Studies reveal the following:

- *Reading* training materials generates about a 10-percent comprehension rate.
- *Hearing* yields a 20-percent comprehension rate.
- *Seeing* increases comprehension to around 30 percent.
- *Watching* someone perform the task brings about 50 percent comprehension.
- Actually *participating* in the task produces a 70-percent comprehension rate.
- And *doing* the actual task or performing a simulation alone results in a 90-percent comprehension rate.

Early Morning Huddles

62

An early morning huddle refers to a mini staff meeting, typically five to 10 minutes in length, held at the start of the business day. Among the purposes:

- To review the highlights of the previous day, including what went particularly well and any compliments heard about staff members, doctors, or the hospital in general. This discussion starts the day on a positive, upbeat note.
- To organize the day's activities. While most client visits are routine, there are unique situations that may require special handling or cause major time delays. Plan ahead: "Mrs. Gumby is coming in at 11. Let's really try to make her smile." Do any of today's clients have payments that are long overdue? If so, who will deal with the matter?
- To learn if anyone needs help with anything on the day's schedule. You'll create an atmosphere of cooperation and problem solve before the need actually arises.

Among the benefits of early morning huddles:

- They eliminate "surprises" (the avoidable ones anyway).
- They improve hospital efficiency and client relations.
- They foster teamwork.

Those who hold early morning huddles are enthusiastic about them. Once the habit is developed, the day seems strangely empty without one.

Is a Counteroffer the Answer?

63

The dilemma: A key employee gives notice that she is leaving to take another job for more money. Do you make a counteroffer to persuade her to stay?

In speaking with veterinarians and hospital managers, the consensus seems to be: No. The reason: The problems caused by counteroffers often outweigh the benefits. For example, if concessions are made and the employee stays, it may lead to resentment among other employees who feel they too deserve a raise, additional perks, change in work schedule, or whatever. Worse yet, a counteroffer to a departing employee may lead to a chain reaction, prompting other employees to use the same tactic to gain concessions.

In addition, if the departing employee has repeatedly asked for a raise and been denied it, she may resent the lengths to which she had to go to get it. At the same time, the practice owner may resent having to make such concessions under duress. Resentment on either side, let alone on *both sides,* is sure to erode employer-employee relations and the spirit of teamwork so necessary in a successful practice.

The one exception: a key employee who is critical to the day-to-day operation of the practice. In the long run, it may cost more to *replace* the person than to *retain* him or her. Consider making a counteroffer in such a case, and take a chance that the aftermath will be smooth sailing.

Exit Interviews

64

Are you simply saying goodbye to departing employees? If so, you are losing an opportunity to obtain valuable feedback about your practice that current employees may be reluctant to provide.

Departing employees tend to speak freely because the fear of reprisal is gone. The exit interview, commonly used in industry, is an excellent means for learning what personnel and operational problems, if any, exist.

Exit interviews are recommended for all departing employees whether they are leaving voluntarily or are fired. In the case of a disgruntled employee, the benefit of an exit interview is that it often can clear the air by clarifying the real circumstances of the employee's departure and bringing about an amicable separation.

Exit interviews are best done in person (rather than with a printed questionnaire) and on a voluntary basis, with 20 to 30 minutes allotted for the conversation. The following questions typically are used for exit interviews. Choose those most appropriate to your circumstances and practice needs:

- Were the employee's salary and benefits about right or less than expected or desired?
- What do you think of the hospital environment? Are changes needed in the work area? The heating and air-conditioning? The lighting? The rest room facilities?
- Did you feel overworked, underutilized, or given the

proper workload? Was the work challenging and interesting? If not, why? Did you experience job-related stress? It so, why?

- Were you reasonably happy at work? Were you satisfied with the job? Did you feel a sense of pride about the practice? Is the hospital a nice place to work? Would you recommend it to others?
- Are other employees happy in their jobs? If not, what are the major complaints, and do you have suggestions for improvement? If you were in charge, what changes would you make?
- Did you like your co-workers? Did you get along with others? Was there a sense of teamwork? A friendly atmosphere? If not, why?
- Do the employees here need new or different office or clinical equipment? Additional training? More or less supervision? More involvement with decisions affecting their work?
- Did I do anything that made your job harder?

Caution: Don't accept everything you're told in an exit interview as necessarily accurate or objective. Departing employees may, for obvious reasons, have an ax to grind and may be vindictive toward another employee—or toward you.

Exit interviews may help you identify problems, learn what remedial action is needed, and reduce the costs and turmoil of employee turnover. They're certainly better than just saying goodbye.

Maintain Alumni Relations

65

Rather than lose touch with former staff members, Phillip E. Bly, a dentist in Indianapolis, started an alumni-relations program so employees who've shared work experiences over the years can stay in touch. He coordinates periodic get-togethers of current and former staff members; the group usually meets for a luncheon in a private dining room at a local country club or hotel. On other occasions, the employees and their spouses gather for a picnic, a swim, bowling, or a Christmas party.

The get-togethers, Dr. Bly reports, are fun—and they provide some unexpected fringe benefits to his practice. For example:

- Most of the former employees remain with the practice as clients.
- Many continue to be active referral sources for the practice.
- On occasion, when Dr. Bly is short-handed, the former employees fill in on an emergency basis—and are glad to help out. In fact, some of them say that being back in the practice is like "old home week."

Although not all of your former employees will want or be able to attend such alumni activities, many will. Those who do will benefit from the ongoing relationships.

Upward Appraisal

66

A Texas veterinarian used to think his employees considered him easy-going. He's since learned they're terrified of him. A Florida hospital manager who thought of herself as efficient discovered that staff members think she's a control freak. Needless to say, neither perceived management style is conducive to employee morale, motivation, and productivity—let alone practice growth.

These people learned about their management styles through what's known as "upward appraisal"—a process by which employees evaluate their managers, and managers learn how staff members perceive their day-to-day behavior and management style.

As you consider an upward appraisal, keep in mind that never hearing complaints about yourself doesn't mean there aren't any. Most employees are understandably timid about giving negative feedback to their boss; others believe it wouldn't change a thing and might cause resentment, if not repercussions. So they talk among themselves, their families, and perhaps among clients about what bothers them about the practice. And the problems continue.

Regardless of the outcome, an upward appraisal will be an adventure in self-discovery that can make you a better manager. To get started, consider the following evaluation form. Use it as is or modify it to suit your needs. Then distribute it to everyone on your staff, emphasizing that no signatures or hand-written answers are required. That will encourage your staff to tell it like it is. *Continued*

Evaluation Form

Doctor _____

Hospital Manager_____

Circle One

1. Personal appearance	1 2 3 4 x
2. Conducts himself/herself in a professional manner	1 2 3 4 x
3. Has a likable personality	1 2 3 4 x
4. Is a good listener	1 2 3 4 x
5. Is good at giving feedback to others	1 2 3 4 x
6. Is open to other people's ideas and opinions	1 2 3 4 x
7. Is thoughtful and considerate of staff members	1 2 3 4 x
8. Looks for win-win solutions to disagreements	1 2 3 4 x
9. Has good self-control when under pressure	1 2 3 4 x
10. Will admit it or apologize when wrong	1 2 3 4 x
11. Is punctual	1 2 3 4 x
12. Leaves personal affairs at home	1 2 3 4 x
13. Is good at giving compliments and positive feedback	1 2 3 4 x
14. Provides on-the-job training	1 2 3 4 x
15. Willingly answers questions of staff members	1 2 3 4 x
16. Makes me proud to work in this practice	1 2 3 4 x
17. Lets me know in a fair and constructive manner when I have done something wrong	1 2 3 4 x
18. Keeps his or her promise	1 2 3 4 x
19. Delegates the authority I need to do my job	1 2 3 4 x
20. Has good people skills	1 2 3 4 x

Signature not required. Use reverse side for comments.

Upward appraisals not only enable you to see yourself as others do, they define and promote an internal code of behavior for all employees (e.g., being punctual, a good listener, thoughtful, and considerate of others). It's saying in effect: This is what our practice is all about.

Hard-Learned Lessons about Personnel Management and Motivation

67

Here's some food for thought as you work to improve your relationship with your staff:

- The question most frequently asked by managers is: "How do I get my employees to do what I want them to do?" A better question: How do I get my employees to *want* to do what I want them to do?
- Trying to motivate others without understanding their motivational needs is like trying to start a stalled car by kicking it.
- People's performance and productivity tend to improve when they know what's expected of them and receive periodic feedback about their work. Action step: Conduct performance reviews.
- The first law of human behavior: Behavior that's rewarded tends to be repeated. Action step: Catch people in the act of doing something right—and tell them so. Corollary: Good work that goes unnoticed and unappreciated tends to deteriorate, almost without exception.
- Studies show that people generate 70 to 80 percent more ideas in a group setting than when thinking alone. Action step: Hold interactive staff meetings.
- It's crazy to lead the band and play all the instruments. Action step: Delegate. *Continued*

If you gave every employee a $1,000 raise starting tomorrow, how much harder would they work—and for how long?

- People labor more diligently to accomplish goals and objectives when they've been allowed to participate in establishing them. Action step: Practice participative management.
- The competence of most people is increased when they are presented with a challenge. Action step: Provide opportunities for employees to s-t-r-e-t-c-h; that is— learn and grow on the job.
- Very few people get the praise they believe they deserve.
- Some people would rather have the *praise* than a *raise*.
- Money motivates people—but only up to a point.
- The way you treat your employees is the way they will treat your clients.
- It isn't the people you fire who make your life miserable, it's the people you *don't fire*.

7

Market Research

The end product of market research is *information,* the fuel for all decision-making about your practice. Among its purposes, market research helps you identify:

- what you and your staff are doing *right*
- what, if anything, you are doing *wrong*
- what changes, if any, are needed.

Blind Spots

68

In the back of the eye where the optic nerve enters, there is an area about 1.5 millimeters in diameter called the blind spot. What makes it unusual is that it is not affected by light and has no sensation of vision. To experience the blind spot, hold this page at arm's length, close your left eye, and look directly at the dot on the left. Then bring the page slowly towards your face. When the page is about 10 to 12 inches away, the right dot will suddenly vanish from view—only to reappear as you bring the page still closer.

●   ●

Blind spots—those things that doctors or staff members unconsciously say or do that turn off clients—also occur in practice management. A few examples:

- a long wait on the telephone
- an ill-humored receptionist
- hospital smells
- an uncommunicative doctor.

If it annoys clients and you're unaware of it, it's a blind spot. And because clients seldom, if ever, mention problems, they persist, taking their toll on goodwill and practice growth. Avoid getting so caught up in everyday pressures that you completely miss problems that are obvious to others.

What Do Clients Want?

69

What do today's consumers want from the stores they frequent? Here's what Yankelovich Partners, a national market-research firm, found:

Factor	Importance
Reasonable prices	90%
Quality merchandise	89%
Treats customers with respect	76%
Makes it quick and easy to shop	67%
Can always find what I want	64%
Convenient hours	64%
Convenient parking	62%
Pleasant atmosphere	61%
Near where I live or work	60%
I can trust prices	56%
Knowledgeable salespeople	52%
Holds a lot of sales	47%

As you can see, the respondents ranked "reasonable prices" and "quality merchandise" well ahead of the other 10 factors when deciding where to shop. This finding corroborates other studies that show that today's consumers are value-driven. The "treats customers with respect" factor experienced the sharpest increase over the previous year's study, up by 15 percent; shopping that's "quick and easy" jumped by 5 percent.

When considering these findings in light of your own practice, ask yourself:

- Do my clients hold similar concerns, in the same order
- of importance, when shopping for veterinary services and pet supplies?
- If so, how well does my practice address these concerns?
- How well does my competition address these concerns?
- What changes, if any, do I need to make to give my clients what they want?

Reality check: Independent surveys of pet owners indicate that a high percentage of companion animal OTC products are purchased from supermarkets, pet shops, discount outlets, and drug stores.

Marketing research also indicates that pet owners shop in these places for four main reasons:

1) They don't realize veterinarians offer these products.

2) They don't realize that the *quality* of these products varies greatly and that in many cases the brands carried by veterinarians are *better* than what they will find elsewhere.

3) They are unaware of the many *value-added services* veterinarians provide—including personnel who are thoroughly familiar with these products and who know which ones to use in any given situation and how to use them properly.

4) In many cases, pet owners don't realize the *cost* of such products is the same, and *possibly less*, from their veterinarian.

Not Sure What Clients Want? Ask Them

70

Rather than second-guess what new services or changes your clients would most like to see in your practice, ask them. How? Construct a client survey that begins: "To help us better serve you and your pet, we are considering some changes in our practice. Your preferences and opinions about the following services would be greatly appreciated."

List those changes you're willing to make and/or services you're willing to add, plus any explanation you feel is necessary; for example:

- extended hours (specify the days of the week and the hours you're considering)
- drop off early/pick-up later policy (indicate what fee, if any, will be charged for this "supervised day care")
- house calls (indicate trip fee)
- drive-up service (see Success Secret 19)
- VIP boarding (see Success Secret 21)
- pick-up/drop-off service (see Success Secret 24)
- nutritional counseling
- behavioral counseling
- microchip identification (indicate fee)
- pet adoption
- separate entrances/reception areas for dogs and cats
- a library of training and breeding books, audio and video cassettes, and related reference materials for client loan or purchase.

Tip

Be selective. Consider focusing your survey on your best, most active clients—the ones who spend the most dollars, make the most referrals, or in the case of food animal practice, are the 20 percent of clients who are responsible for 80 percent of your business.

Food Animal Practitioners: Consider the same approach to survey clients about policy changes and/or the addition of new services. For example, you might include:
- producer meetings (including specific topics you and/or an outside speaker would present)
- a client newsletter (with suggested topics such as seasonal tips and technology and research updates).

From the Success File

Dave Richards, DVM, owner of the Animal Health Center in Valdosta, Ga., asked his cat-owning clients the following question: What would this hospital have to provide to persuade you to bring your cats in for lodging when you leave town? ("Lodging," Dr. Richards says, has a different connotation than "boarding" and helps differentiate his upscale facility from a kennel.)

The consensus? His clients wanted their cats to have "more exercise and a place to look out a window while resting."

In response, Dr. Richards built a playroom for cats with a climbing tree made of four-inch polyvinyl chloride pipe covered with carpeting; he also added an exterior window with a wide ledge—purr-fect for sleeping in the sun.

The result: Revenues from cat lodging increased dramatically.

Learn from Clients' Experiences

71

Some clients volunteer the reason they left their previous veterinarian. Others remain closed-mouth about it.

When you don't know the reason, you and your staff are in the dark as to what, if anything, went wrong—and how you might prevent it from happening in your practice. Of course, if the client moved away from the area or some other such reason, it's a closed matter. But suppose it was because the previous veterinarian:
- "never explained anything"
- "was always rushed"
- "was indignant when I wanted a second opinion."

Or in the case of food animal practice:
- "was too slow to come to the farm after I called"
- "either didn't care about my records or didn't know what to do with them."

With such information, you'd *know* what the client wanted (or didn't want) and you and your staff could accommodate him or her.

Action step: Consider saying to new clients, "If you don't mind my asking, could you please tell me the reason you left your previous veterinarian? If there were problems of any kind, I want to make sure they don't happen here."

Some clients will hesitate to tell you the reason, perhaps masking the fact that they left owing a lot of money. How-

Marketing Myopia

Not knowing the reason(s) new clients left their previous veterinarian —then unintentionally repeating the same blunder.

ever, some clients will gladly answer that question to avoid a repeat of the same problems. Of course, there also will be clients who say they really liked, perhaps loved, their previous veterinarian and truly regretted having to leave his or her practice. If appropriate, inquire as to the reasons for their affection and loyalty.

Variation: If you're not comfortable with this approach, consider asking new clients more general questions about their experiences with other veterinarians. Have they been positive or negative—and why? The information you obtain from such inquiries will greatly accelerate the process of bonding new clients to your practice.

From the Success File

To make sure clinicians at the University of Missouri Veterinary Teaching Hospital address the chief concerns of clients coming to their facility, a brief questionnaire is given to clients when they arrive. The first question: "In order of decreasing importance to you, list the reasons (or symptoms or services desired) for today's visit," followed by ample space for clients' answers. This way, clinicians and clients are, as they say, on the same page.

Client Retention

The average practice loses 10 to 30 percent of its clients each year and unfortunately you can't assume that a client who doesn't complain isn't upset; often angry clients just quietly leave your practice.

On those occasions when such a client *announces* his or her departure, or when by chance you or a staff member learn of it, consider sending the following letter:

I'm sorry to learn that you've decided to leave our practice. If our team has failed to meet your expectations in any way, we'd like to know about it—and have another chance. If we can be of service to you at any time in the future, please don't hesitate to call us. (This sentence leaves the door open in case clients find the quality of care and service they receive elsewhere to be unsatisfactory.)

There are two main reasons clients decide to leave:

• The veterinary team fails to meet their expectations.
• The veterinary team mismanages a critical "moment of truth." (See Success Secret 32.)

If there's room for forgiveness, this low-key letter may convince the client you've earned another chance.

72

Reality Check

If a letter such as that described here could retrieve only one or two clients who made the decision to leave your practice, it would be well worth the effort.

73

"No Holds Barred" Staff Meeting

A low-cost way to undertake market research and identify your practice's strengths and weaknesses is to ask your staff. Staff members frequently hear clients' comments about the practice, but they seldom share such information. Why? Because the doctors with whom they work never ask.

To tap into this resource, distribute a list of questions to your staff, then schedule a "no-holds barred" meeting to discuss their responses. Sample questions include:

- What compliments about the practice do you hear most often?
- What complaints do you frequently hear?
- Where, when, and why do misunderstandings with clients most frequently occur, and what are your recommendations for solving these misunderstandings?
- What changes will improve client satisfaction?

Staff members tend to be more objective about the practice than the doctors. Plus, they view the clients from a different perspective and see and hear things the doctors don't. Listen to their ideas and insights—they may open your eyes to opportunities for improving client satisfaction and practice growth.

Focus Groups

74

Long used in qualitative market research about consumer products, focus groups are beginning to be used by veterinarians to view their practices through the eyes of their clients. A typical focus group consists of eight to 10 invited clients who meet for one to 1-1/2 hours to talk specifically about the practice.

The ideal focus-group participant is astute, verbal, and willing to speak up about the practice—for better or worse. The setting can be the hospital itself in the evening or an off-site location such as a restaurant. Light refreshments are typically served. Participants are sometimes paid a token amount; the average is $25.

Some doctors hire a professional focus-group facilitator, who, by definition, is neutral about the practice and more likely to make the participants comfortable enough to express their true feelings. To locate such a facilitator, contact the business school at a local college, where a professor or a graduate student may be available. Other doctors utilize a hospital manager or staff member who has the skills to start the discussion and then listen without interrupting or becoming defensive.

To start the discussion, consider asking the participants the following types of questions:

- In your experience with the practice, what have you liked? What have you disliked?
- Can you think of specific situations you wish the staff

Variation

Want more cat owners in your practice? Equine clients? Thirty-five- to 50-year-old career people? Breeders? Consider focus groups consisting only of clients from each of these or other constituencies. Each group will have its own point of view, likes and dislikes.

had handled differently? What about situations the doctor could have handled differently?

- Why did you choose this veterinary hospital above all others? (See Success Secret 75.)
- How do you feel about the hospital environment? Could it be improved? How about the hospital's hours? Appointment scheduling? Selection of animal health-care products?

Ralph Waldo Emerson said: "The field cannot be seen from within the field." Focus groups are one of numerous market-research techniques that can help you get that all-important outside view of your practice—through the eyes of your clients.

Why Clients Chose Your Practice Above All Others

75

Many veterinarians don't know for sure why clients chose their practice above all others in the community. Some "think" they know or can "guess" all the reasons. Others "hope" it is for the reasons they *want* to be the reasons. And some haven't a clue as to what those reasons are.

Without knowing the actual reasons clients choose your practice, you leave long-range planning for your practice to guesswork, trial and error, and intuition—all of which may miss the mark. For example, one veterinarian moved his companion animal practice to a new location "only" seven miles away, believing his clients would gladly follow him. What he failed to realize was how important the former location was to his clients—most of whom *did not* follow him.

The point is: If one of the reasons that clients most frequently mention for choosing your practice is location or early morning appointments or reasonable fees, don't be quick to make a change—assuming you want to retain your current client base.

76

Is Yellow Pages Advertising a Good Investment?

Most veterinarians who advertise in the yellow pages are doing so to attract new clients, jump-start a new or sluggish practice, or replace clients lost to the competition. Is such advertising a good investment?

There are several considerations. One is cost. For example, at an annual cost of, say, $6,000, a yellow page display ad would need to produce $24,000 in additional revenue just to break even (assuming a profit margin of 25 percent). To achieve that increase with an average client transaction charge of $50, a practice would need to see 480 new clients a year, or an average of 40 a month. Substitute your own numbers to determine the requirements for your advertising to pay for itself.

Another consideration: Other veterinary practices with larger, more attention-getting display ads in the same directory will decrease the effectiveness of yours—and perhaps completely overshadow it.

If you're considering a display ad in the yellow pages (or if you have one and wonder how well it's working), screen new clients by asking how they *first* learned about your practice. The word "first" is critical. Oddly enough, many clients will say they learned about your practice from the yellow pages, when in fact, it was only where they found your address and telephone number. With further probing, you may learn they *first* heard about your practice from a friend, a pet shop owner, or someone else who spoke highly of you.

In my company, we find that after veterinarians track the number of new clients and how clients first learned about their practices, many discontinue yellow pages advertising—and suffer little if any drop in the numbers of new clients. What most conclude is that word-of-mouth referrals are their best and most cost-effective source of new clients.

Engage an Outside Firm

77

To learn what their dairy clients think of the quality of their services, the price of those services, and what changes or improvements are needed, a multi-doctor practice in the Midwest engaged an outside firm to conduct a survey.

To encourage complete candor, the survey form assured clients, "Your responses will not be seen by the doctors or the staff and there is no way your survey form can be personally identified."

Clients responded to a series of statements using a 1 (strongly disagree) to 10 (strongly agree) scale. Among the statements:

- The time required for the doctors to get to the farm after being called is satisfactory.
- Once on the farm, the doctor is willing to do additional, unscheduled procedures.
- The appearance and cleanliness of the veterinarians and the vehicles are satisfactory.
- I feel I get what I pay for.
- The veterinarian appears interested in the health of my animals.
- Treatments prescribed are adequately discussed.
- I approve of veterinary school students accompanying the veterinarian on farm calls.
- I would like to see additional procedures and equipment added to the practice.

Clients also were asked to complete the following statements:

- The thing I like most about the practice is …
- The thing I would most like to see changed at the practice is …
- An additional service I would like the practice to provide is …

Clients' responses proved overwhelmingly favorable, but they did express a few concerns about emergency service, response time, the telephone answering service, communications with veterinarians during non-business hours, and certain high-profile fees.

As the renowned educator John Dewey observed, a problem well-stated is half-solved. The tragedy occurs when problems go undetected, taking their toll in the loss of client goodwill and referrals—and sometimes the clients themselves.

78

The Post-Appointment Telephone Interview

Tip

As in any interview, the more you draw the person out the more you'll learn. The use of what psychologists call "attentive noises," such as "hmmm," "aha" and "ahh" send a signal that you are interested in what the other person is saying and you want him or her to continue.

A follow-up interview with a client can be a valuable marketing-research tool. Choose 10 or 15 clients who represent a cross-section of your client base to call and interview; two or three days after an appointment is an ideal time to get feedback. To sensitize everyone on your team to the importance of client satisfaction, rotate this duty among staff members.

To expedite the interviews, ask a staff member to make arrangements with the pre-selected clients at the conclusion of their hospital visits. For example:

Mrs. Carlson, we plan to call a few of the clients we see this week to ask about their experience while visiting our hospital. We'd very much like your opinion on this subject. Would you be willing to be interviewed for just a few minutes later this week at a time that is convenient for you?

Most clients are willing—if not flattered—to be interviewed and will indicate a preferred day or time to be called. Among the questions you might ask:

- How did everything go during your visit?
- Were all of your questions answered?
- Was there anything big or small that bothered you?
- Is there anything we could have done to make your visit

to our practice a more positive experience?
- If a friend were looking for a veterinarian, would you be comfortable recommending our practice?

An alternative to the post-appointment telephone interview is for the receptionist to ask departing clients: How did everything go today? In asking such a question, it's important to hold eye contact with the client and look genuinely interested. Otherwise, the client may not attach any importance to the question and simply say "fine."

Regardless of what you hear—brickbats or bouquets—the feedback you obtain from such interviews will enable you to identify the goals of market research stated at the beginning of this chapter:

- what you and your staff are doing right
- what, if anything, you are doing wrong
- what changes, if any, are needed.

Notes

8

Fee Strategies

79

Put Fees in Proper Perspective

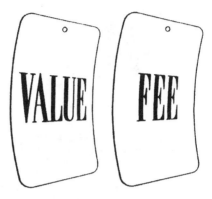

Which of these cards looks bigger: the one with the word "value" or the one with the word "fee"?

Most people say the card with the word fee looks bigger. Actually, the cards are the same size. The fee card *appears* larger because the eyes tend to focus on the center of the picture where the short side of the value card is compared with the long side of the fee card.

When clients complain about being overcharged for veterinary services, they too are not seeing the whole picture. The key to putting fees in perspective is twofold: Provide value-added services, and let clients know what you've done for them.

For example, food animal practitioners can build value by:

- taking the time to walk through a farrowing house, dairy barn, or feedlot to evaluate the housing, degree of confinement, temperature, ventilation, humidity, manure-handling procedures, and related matters;
- studying a client's records on fertility, feed conversion, disease incidence, milk production, and similar performance criteria;
- sitting down with the client to review your findings, diagnosis, and recommendations for a total herd-health program;
- going a step further and preparing a written report that summarizes everything.

Doing more for clients and letting them know the particulars helps them see the entire picture. It makes value the focus of their attention, and puts fees in proper perspective.

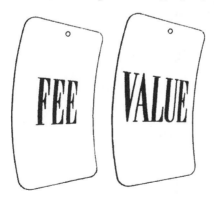

Continued

129

From the Success File

- *The experience of Charles Halford, DVM, owner of the Millington Animal Hospital in Millington, Tenn., proves that price isn't everything. Among the clinics in Millington is a military base veterinary facility that charges approximately one-third of Dr. Halford's fee for canine vaccinations, physical exam, heartworm check, and fecal—yet more than 60 percent of Dr. Halford's clients are military. "We wouldn't be cheap," Dr. Halford says, "so we decided to be nice."*

- *In Clarksville, Tenn., Scott Loxley, DVM, co-owner of the East View Veterinary Clinic, faces similar differences between his fees and those of a nearby veterinary facility on a military base—yet he too sees large numbers of military personnel who prefer the service and personal attention at his clinic.*

Price Isn't Everything

Studies of consumer behavior indicate that only 13 percent of people make buying decisions based strictly on price. The consumers in this small group—either because of circumstances or because they don't know better—always look for the lowest price. That means 87 percent of people consider price—but *also* look for quality, good service, convenience, a personal relationship, and more from their service providers.

Considering the buying potential of each group, does it make sense to gear your practice—and fee structure—to the price-conscious 13 percent of the population? You may drown in overhead costs trying to keep prices low enough to suit them. And by definition, they will leave your practice if they can find lower prices elsewhere.

You may be thinking that more than 13 percent of your community is price-conscious. Perhaps so. But even if you double this number, that leaves 74 percent of people who are interested in factors besides cost—still a sizable target population for your practice. If you tripled the figure to 39 percent, you could still target 61 percent of the population as prospective clients—more than you and your present staff could handle.

You can't be all things to all people, so why not provide the quality of care, personal service, convenience, and one-to-one relationships that meet the needs of the 87 percent to whom price isn't everything?

Reality Check

If price were everything, supermarket shelves would be filled with generic products priced lower than their branded counterparts. As it is, generic products account for only a small fraction of supermarket sales.

The Rule of the Marketplace

81

Reality Check

I recognize that aggressive, hard-selling, low-cost competition can do serious damage to a practice taking the "high road." Flexibility is vital—as Success Secrets 82 and 83 indicate.

Having said "price isn't everything" in Success Secret 80, let me qualify that statement.

Price isn't everything to clients who realize there are differences between a procedure performed at your hospital and one performed at considerably less cost at a competing facility. In addition, clients must believe the difference in patient care and client service is worth the difference in cost. As psychologist William James noted, a difference that makes no difference—is not a difference.

The real problem, as management guru Tom Peters points out, is that "Perception is all there is. There is no reality as such, only *perceived reality.* It's the way each of us chooses to perceive a communication, the quality of a product, or the value of a service."

In the marketplace, perception *is* everything. And it's clients who have the deciding vote. That's the rule of the marketplace.

The good news is that perceptions can be changed. Differentiation, image management, client education, and front-desk service are among the strategies discussed in this book that will do the job.

How to Coexist
with the Superstores

Veterinarians whose retail operations are being adversely affected by the superstore phenomenon may benefit from studies done by Kenneth E. Stone, PhD, an economics professor at Iowa State University. He investigated the repercussions to small retailers of a Wal-Mart store opening in the area. He concluded that it *is* possible for small businesses to compete with superstores—but not without changes in day-to-day operations.

Among his recommendations:

- **Sharpen your pricing skills**. Discount merchandisers focus their price reductions on frequently purchased items—items for which customers comparison-shop. The average customer then assumes that prices on all other items in the store must be lower than they are elsewhere. Conversely, when local businesses charge a higher price than Wal-Mart for the same frequently purchased items, customers infer that everything else in the store is high-priced as well.

  Independent merchants, Professor Stone says, need to identify the items for which customers comparison-shop and make a special effort to keep prices on those items competitive.
- **Emphasize expert technical advice**. It's difficult to find superstore employees who know the merchandise or the customer. This shortcoming gives smaller businesses an

opportunity to build a loyal clientele by helping customers analyze problems and find products to meet their needs.

- **Train your employees.** In the customer's eyes, the employee *is* the business. Training your staff can have one of the highest payoffs of any investment you make.
- **Visit the superstores frequently**. Keep informed of what you're up against.

Business-as-usual is a luxury that few practices can maintain in today's challenging, highly competitive environment.

Market-Driven Pricing

83

If you are losing significant numbers of clients to low-cost vaccination facilities, it may be time to consider a market-driven pricing strategy for vaccinations and other comparison-shopped services. Why? To keep your fees on those items competitive with those of low-cost veterinary providers in your area.

Gary S. Atkinson, DVM, owner of the four-doctor County Animal Hospital in Manchester, Mo., a suburb of St. Louis, is surrounded by numerous discount vaccination facilities. When an increasing number of his established clients began to respond to the facilities' extensive vaccination promotions, Dr. Atkinson sent a letter offering a "no-frills level of service" at considerably lower fees for vaccinations and for heartworm and fecal tests. The physical exam that went with these services became optional.

"The purpose of this vaccination program wasn't to attract new clients," says Jan Eversgerd, the hospital's office manager, "but rather to prevent the loss of existing clients—especially those who believe their pets are healthy and don't want to pay for an exam. And the program," she adds, "has worked."

When a client calls for a "vaccination-only appointment," the records are pulled while the client is on the phone. If the pet is overdue for an exam, the client is advised. Some choose the low-cost alternative; many opt for both the exam and the vaccinations. The important thing, Eversgerd says, "is that they stay in the practice."

Continued

In today's highly competitive, cost-conscious environment, client retention can be the key to survival. Market-driven pricing is one of many strategies that can help you achieve it.

From the Success File

Richard Thomas, DVM, owner of the nine-doctor Animal Medical and Surgical Hospital in Irving, Texas, admits he fell victim to a mistake practitioners commonly make.

"In 1989," he recalls, "a mobile vaccination facility began operations directly across the street from our hospital. A nationally known pet superstore also opened nearby. Both heavily advertised low-cost vaccinations.

"I refused to compete on price," he continues, "believing my clients would never choose such services based solely on price. I was wrong. In their minds, vaccinations were a com-modity. And our vaccination revenues plunged by over 70 percent.

"If I could replay the situation," he says, "I would match any price on service. You don't have to beat *their prices, just match them. I'd also create a niche in the market that the competitors* couldn't *provide. And I'd get to know my clients better. That's what we're doing now. And the clients are coming back."*

Clarify Before You Explain or Compromise

84

You quote a fee to a client. The client replies, "That's a lot of money," or words to that effect. How do you respond?

The veterinarians and staff members I've interviewed respond in a variety of ways. Some become angry. Some deny that the procedure is expensive. Some defend and justify their fees. Others are quick to offer extended payment options, or a less-costly alternative. In many cases, these explanations and compromises are premature—if not totally inappropriate.

The first step in such a situation is to clarify what the client is really saying. For example, "that's a lot of money" could mean any of the following:

- It's not worth it.
- It's more than I paid the last time.
- It's more than I saw advertised by another facility.
- It's more than I can afford at this time.
- I never dreamt this would be so expensive.
- How am I ever going to explain this to my spouse?

Each of these underlying meanings requires an entirely different response. A simple, follow-up question asked in a sincere manner may be all that's needed. For example, you might ask: "Why do you say that's a lot of money?"

When you know what the objection really is, you are in a position to address it.

Reality Check

You may be surprised to learn that some clients won't have a reason for saying or implying, "that's a lot of money." In many cases, it's just a knee-jerk reaction to a higher fee than they had in mind. In such cases, a defensive or flip response such as "Isn't Fluffy worth it?" is uncalled for, inappropriate, and in the words of one client, "equivalent to emotional blackmail."

85

How to Handle Complaints About Fees

Word Magic

I've asked countless veterinarians for their response to the client who says: "I pay you more than I pay my own doctor." The best response I've heard came from Don Ward, DVM, of Tampa, Fla., who merely said, "I hope you always do!"

Do clients ever complain about fees? Ask you to lower them? Compare them with lower fees advertised by others? Here's one way to respond:

> *"Our fees are based on a number of factors: the time involved, the level of skill required, the number of services provided, the caliber of people who work with me, our facilities and equipment, the continuing education of all staff members, and the quality of drugs used. If we were to reduce fees, I'd have to leave something out. And frankly, I don't know what to eliminate without compromising our service."*

This explanation is even more meaningful if clients have actually experienced or already know about these elements of your fees. Hospital tours, practice brochures, itemized bills, and explanations of the services you and your staff provide all make clients more aware and appreciative of what's involved—and more inclined to pay your fees cheerfully and promptly.

Suppose a client *doesn't* accept the logic of this response and again compares your fee with a lower fee quoted or advertised by another veterinary facility? Consider this approach:

There are others who will do this procedure for less. The problem with having it done elsewhere is that you don't get me, my staff, and our concern for your pet before, during, and after the surgery. We're an integral part of the package.

I can understand your concern for cost. You'll have to decide what's most important to you.

Such a statement gives the client something other than cost to think about.

Itemize Services Performed

86

Tip

Don Polley, DVM, owner of the Harvester Animal Clinic in St. Charles, Mo., lists three levels of dental cleaning: routine, intermediate, and extensive. Each is based on the degree of disease present and is charged for accordingly.

Do clients ever complain that it costs more to have their dog's teeth cleaned than it does for their own? What such clients don't realize is that in addition to the thorough cleaning their dog's teeth received, there also may have been lab tests to determine anesthetic safety, the anesthesia itself, and perhaps antibiotics—none of which are used routinely in human dentistry.

To put fees in proper perspective, itemize the component services performed. The two common ways to do so are to present fees as *bundled* (list the services performed and show only a total fee at the bottom), or unbundled (assign a separate charge to each component service).

If any services or products are provided at no charge, include them on the itemized bill and mark them "no charge." Doing so will enhance their perceived value.

Outlining the many steps of each procedure will help clients appreciate the *value* of your professional services.

From the Success File

Jan Bellows, DVM, Dipl. AVDC, of Pembroke Pines, Fla., went a step further by creating a client handout that itemizes fees for each procedure. For example, the "dental fee sheet" itemizes periodontal therapy to include root planing, curettage, fluoride treatment, apical reposition surgery, and guided tissue regeneration. Extraction and endodontic fees are based on the number of roots involved.

Itemize and Explain

At the Veterinary Medical Clinic in Tampa, Fla., a "medical waste disposal fee" is charged for cases involving surgery and/or the use of syringes, needles, or X-rays. The explanation on the invoice states:

> Because of new environmental protection laws, there is a $1.10 environmental impact fee charged to each pet that is treated to comply with the environmental regulations required to dispose of hazardous materials.

Clinic Director Eddie Garcia, DVM, emphasizes that the $1.10 fee is per case, regardless of the number of procedures performed. "Clients consider the charge to be reasonable," he says, "and acceptance has been excellent."

Another option: Alan F. Berger, DVM, owner of Macomb Veterinary Associates, in Utica, Mich., itemizes a dental cleaning in terms of the *time* it takes:

> An average dental cleaning (dogs, cats, ferrets) at Macomb Veterinary Associates takes 6 minutes to establish and stabilize the inhalation anesthesia; 16 minutes to remove the tartar by hand and/or by ultrasonic methods; and 21 minutes to skillfully polish every tooth. 'Economy' dentistry often omits the first and last steps."   *Continued*

87

Reality Check

"Most client complaints about fees that are received by AAHA and other veterinary organizations deal with failures in communication about the fees charged, rather than the amount actually charged for the services."

—The 1995 AAHA Report: A Study Of The Companion Animal Veterinary Services Market, Page 125

In addition to the standard charges for pre-operative and surgical procedures, Gary Dehne, DVM, owner of the Walnut Hill Animal Hospital in Gaithersburg, Md., includes on the bill an "operating room fee" as follows:

- OR minimum (for procedures taking 10 minutes or less)
- OR^1 (10 to 30 minutes)
- OR^2 (30 to 45 minutes)
- OR^3 (45 minutes or more)

"In cases where clients have objected to a bill," Dr. Dehne says, "the operating room fee has not been criticized."

The High-Fee Paradox

88

Periodic fee increases do cause some price-conscious clients to leave a practice—although veterinarians invariably report that fewer clients leave than they anticipated. What's interesting, though, is that about 10 to 15 percent of practices actually *get busier* following an increase in fees. Research indicates three reasons for this paradox:

1) Most veterinarians who charge more for a given procedure *try harder* to provide above-average patient care and client service, which in turn delights clients and leads to more referrals and a busier practice.

2) Charging higher fees that clients cheerfully and promptly pay boosts self-confidence, makes veterinary medicine more satisfying, and has a positive impact on patient care, client services, and practice growth.

3) As mentioned earlier, people tend to judge the unknown (quality of service) by the known (fees)—and fees do have an impact on the image of a veterinary practice. It's not scientific, but it's the way some people think. It also helps explain the high fee paradox or why "low-price" advertising turns some people off. They figure "there must be a catch." And often, they're right.

Do these findings mean that you should raise your fees no matter what? Definitely not. There are numerous other factors to consider. The high-fee paradox, however, is a marketplace phenomenon worth noting.

89

If You Hate Discussing Fees with Clients ...

Warning

Make sure the person to whom you are delegating fee discussions and collections doesn't hate these tasks as much as you do. Sky-high accounts receivable may result.

Tip

Screen job applicants for this position by asking: "How do you feel about asking people for money?"

... you're not alone. Clients who complain that your fees are high are particularly taxing. An increasing number of veterinarians are delegating such discussions to staff members—and reaping great benefits. Among them:

- Most clients, many of whom are women, seem more comfortable discussing fees with a woman—or as one working person to another—than with a doctor, male or female. "Staff members are more understanding," clients say.
- Employees are less likely to make concessions, round off fees, or offer discounts to the doctor's friends. Veterinarians and staff members agree: Total income is higher when staff members make financial arrangements.
- Collections improve when the person making the initial arrangements also is responsible for collections. This policy averts any "He said I shouldn't worry about the bill" type excuses for not paying on time.

To best delegate fee discussions and collections, explain your clinical findings and recommendations to clients, and then refer them to a staff member who can review the costs involved and answer questions. Delegate fee discussions selectively or totally—depending on how much you hate the task.

Supervised Neglect

90

I've observed countless DVM-client interactions in exam rooms throughout the country and reached the following conclusion: The reason more *needed* diagnostic tests and treatment procedures aren't performed isn't because clients decline them, it's because they're not *offered* to clients. The reasons vary. In some cases, veterinarians are making "economic decisions" for their clients; in others, veterinarians simply are taking the path of least resistance.

But consider this: I've spoken with many veterinarians who say that not recommending or even perhaps requiring such services as pre-anesthetic/pre-surgical profiles of older pets is a disservice to the patient and client. In fact, some say it's the equivalent of "supervised neglect"—regardless of the small percentage of abnormal results found in such tests.

Action Step: Be a pet advocate. Give clients a chance to say "no" to the diagnostic tests and treatment procedures that are clinically indicated for their pets. Many veterinarians do so with pre-printed recommendations that clients can authorize or refuse. High percentages are accepting. Also give clients a chance to say "no" to other elective procedures when indicated, such as ECG, X-rays, endoscopy, ultrasonography, thyroid function testing, topical fluoride, and pain medication among numerous others.

When writing a prescription for an ear infection, rather than telling a client, "If Snoopy isn't better in a week, call me," explain the importance of seeing the pet in a week for a brief follow-up visit. Then either recommend that the client make an appointment before leaving or ask the receptionist to book a follow-up visit. The worst that will happen? The client will say "no."

From the Success File

Janet Buck, RVT, hospital manager at Graber's Animal Hospital in Toledo, Ohio, reports 75 percent client acceptance of such re-check visits, which are charged at a reduced office visit fee.

Hard-Learned Lessons about Fees

91

Review this list when reviewing the fees in your practice:

- Make *clinical* decisions for clients—not *economic* decisions. Reason: You can't X-ray clients' pocketbooks or ascertain what they're willing to pay or can afford.
- The two-word formula to reduce complaints about fees: *no surprises.* Inform before you perform.
- Charge clients for what you do based on your overhead, time, and expertise. Especially your expertise.
- I've seen more practices hurt by fees that were *too low* than I have by fees that were *too high.*
- Don't let your most price-sensitive clients govern your fee structure.
- Low fees combined with high volume and high overhead are a formula for grossing yourself to death.
- Another problem with low fees: They tend to attract clients who, by definition, are going to leave your practice if they find lower fees elsewhere.
- There always will be someone willing to do what you do at a lower fee.
- To a client who says, "I don't want to spend a lot of money on this …," consider replying, "I'll tell you what needs to be done, then you decide."
- If you never get complaints about fees, it means either: (1) you and your staff are providing high-quality care and first-rate service—and your clients think it's worth

every penny, or (2) you're undercharging.

- Ask your staff how often clients remark after seeing the bill, "Is that all? I thought it would be a lot more!"
- Don't apologize for fees. Doing so plants the seed that you lack confidence or that your fee is exorbitant. It may even be construed as an invitation to "bargain" for a lower fee.
- It doesn't make sense to provide clinical excellence and charge for mediocrity.
- The key to long-term practice growth is *revenue enhancement*—not *cost containment*.
- High fees rarely scare clients away; low fees rarely bring them in. In fact, sometimes they have the opposite effect.
- When you raise fees, should you give clients advance notice? Write letters with explanations about escalating costs? Post bulletin-board notices? The consensus of veterinarians with whom I've spoken: Just do it!
- Remember: If you do raise fees, you're under no obligation to maintain them. If there are signs of significant client resistance, you can and possibly should reduce fees to their previous levels. But work the numbers first. Sometimes, less is more.
- In all the years I've been surveying veterinarians on the subject, I've met only a handful who raised their fees and later regretted it.

Stress Management

The Lessons of the Slow-Moving Line

92

The place: Myrtle Beach, S.C. I'd flown there from New York via Atlanta. The trip seemed longer than it was, and I was hot, tired, and anxious to get a night's rest. When I got to the hotel, there were perhaps five or six people waiting in line to check in. I joined them. The line inched along. Ten minutes later, it seemed as though I had hardly moved, yet no one was complaining.

"There aren't that many people in line," I thought. "Why is this taking so long?" Finally, I reached the registration desk and was cheerfully greeted by a young clerk. On her coat jacket was a small badge that read: "I'm new—but I'm trying."

The mystery of the slow-moving line was solved. My mood changed. I started to laugh.

"This crowd giving you a hard time?" I asked.

"Not at all," she replied. "Everyone's been so patient and understanding."

I knew why.

I learned two lessons from this incident: 1. Perhaps such a badge would make a new job less stressful for an inexperienced person who doesn't move quite as fast as some clients would like; and 2. Many management problems can be made less troublesome if you think about them creatively.

A High
Tolerance for Contact

93

Part of your job and even more so, your *employees'* jobs, involves what sociologist Arlie Hochschild calls "emotional labor." The term refers to work in which cheerfulness, warmth, sympathetic concern, and the like are an important part of job performance—and *expected* by the clients with whom you and your staff interact.

Having to display such emotions with one client after another, day after day, whether you're up to the task or not, is taxing—especially if clients are distraught, impatient, demanding, unappreciative, or otherwise unhappy about being in your hospital in the first place.

Above all, such repetitive encounters require what's called a "high tolerance for contact." People who lack this trait find it uncomfortable and psychologically draining to deal with client after client. They can become moody, irritable, and even hostile toward clients. Needless to say, this situation takes its toll on client relations and practice growth.

If you do not have a high tolerance for contact, the simplest remedy is to surround yourself with staff members who do.

Stress-Proof Your Practice

94

Stressed-out employees are disruptive to everyone in a veterinary practice. These individuals are often tardy, inefficient, careless, and demoralizing to co-workers and clients. Although some sources of stress in an employee's life, such as divorce, a family member's illness, and so on, are beyond your control, there are some stressful elements of the work environment you can control. For example:

- **Role overload**. It's not uncommon to hear employees say: "There's just too much work to do and never enough time. I don't know where to start."
- **Role conflict**. Are you sending mixed messages? For example, do you instruct employees to be friendly and helpful to clients, while, at the same time, expecting them to handle an increasing number of clients and patients, phone calls, and paperwork? If a bottleneck occurs, which "role" takes precedence?
- **Role ambiguity**. When employees are uncertain about exactly what is expected of them on a day-to-day basis, they experience stress. "My job has not turned out to be the way it was described to me when I was hired" is a common complaint.

How do you control these stressful workplace situations? By developing detailed, written job descriptions that spell out what is expected of each employee. If job descriptions already exist, review, and update them, and prioritize each task. You also might consider job responsibility trade-offs between employees, or hiring additional, part-time employees to alleviate the work load of your full-time staff members.

For job descriptions to be successful, you must obtain one-on-one input from employees and, if appropriate, negotiate any differences in your mutual expectations. Happy, stress-free employees pave the way to client satisfaction and practice growth.

From the Success File

The best guideline I've heard for staffing a client-focused, service-driven, high-performance practice comes from Robert T. Moore, DVM, of Wilson, N.C., who says, "We're staffed for the busiest times; not the slowest." Combined with written job descriptions, his approach eliminates the problems of role overload, conflict, and ambiguity. At the same time, it ensures top-notch service—at all times.

95

Adding a Sense of Fun to Your Practice

Tip

You don't have to be elaborate. Fun activities need only provide a change of pace, a way to unwind if only for a few minutes, a way to celebrate and appreciate each other.
The mood of the practice is important. If your practice is an upbeat place to be, your clients and patients will respond better— and you and your staff will be better for it.

There are some serious benefits to adding a sense of fun to the work environment. David Abramis, Ph.D., of California State University's School of Business Administration, has shown that employees who find fun in their work report that they are more satisfied with their work and lives in general, more motivated by their work, more creative, better able to meet job demands, and less likely to be late for work.

The following are a few ideas I've seen used to generate a sense of fun in veterinary practices:

- **"Goodies."** Everyone brings homegrown, homemade, or store-bought food to work on a rotating basis. In many cases, there's a budget established for the purpose. Snack food is fun and promotes camaraderie.
- **In-hospital lunches.** Great for staff meetings, celebrations, and bad weather days.
- **Bulletin boards.** Post jokes, cartoons, and perhaps photographs of staff members and doctors as infants (a great guessing game for waiting clients).
- **Celebrations.** Help celebrate birthdays, employment anniversaries, going away, or "welcome aboard" occasions, or "just because parties"—with gag gifts.
- **Designated days.** Anyone making a negative remark is fined 25 cents, which goes into a fund for fun occasions.

Instant Vacations

96

In the first century A.D., Phaedrus said, "You will break the bow if you keep it always stretched." He might well have been referring to the importance of what I call "instant vacations." These are spur-of-the-moment breaks during such non-stop, highly focused activity as back-to-back client visits or multiple surgeries. Numerous studies confirm that the rested body is more successful and more productive than a tired one.

Ben Hara, a busy podiatric surgeon in Covina, Calif., routinely takes instant vacations in the form of mid-day naps following a simple lunch. During this time, there are no phone calls, no visitors, no interruptions of any kind. "My mid-day nap," he says, "re-energizes me, increases my productivity, enables me to make two days out of one."

Here's another relaxation technique: Sit or lie down in a comfortable place. Close your eyes. Become aware of your breathing. Breathe in through the nose to a count of four. Exhale through the mouth to a count of four. Picture a mountain meadow. Hear the rushing water. See the wild flowers. Feel the breeze. Hear the sounds of birds. With every intruding thought, repeat the phrase, "I am thinking of a mountain meadow." Do this exercise for 10 minutes, using a timer if necessary.

Other techniques include meditation, autohypnosis, progressive relaxation, and biofeedback. Consider using one to give yourself an instant vacation. You'll discover the benefits far outweigh the small loss of time.

Emotional Economics

97

I am indebted to Harriette and Bill Carney, DVM, Meridian, Miss., for the provocative phrase "emotional economics." It refers to the dilemma of whether it's worth the time, money, and stress to deal with the handful of clients who are unreasonable, demanding, and/or unappreciative of you and your staff's best efforts. You know the kind—clients who are forever complaining and whom there is no pleasing.

There are basically two solutions to this dilemma: 1. If the emotional costs and economic benefits are worth it, grin and bear it; 2. If not, consider dismissing the client. Mrs. Carney suggests something along the following lines: "I want to apologize to you. Apparently we are unable to serve you in a manner that pleases you. Under the circumstances, it might be best for you to seek care for Fluffy at another clinic that can better suit your needs. If you do so, please have them call us and we will provide a vaccination history."

Practitioners tell me they get a variety of reactions to "dismissing" a client. Some animal owners realize they've been out of line, apologize for their behavior, and become model clients. Others take the hint and leave, destined to harass other practices.

Either way, you and your staff win.

The Drive to Achieve

98

One of the questions I'm frequently asked is "How do I motivate my partner (or associate) to work harder (or faster or take more entrepreneurial interest in the practice)?"

At the onset, it's important to recognize that the drive to achieve is not uniformly distributed. Your style may be to keep pushing for more clients and practice growth, no matter what it takes. When you arrive at some pre-determined goal, it probably seems perfectly natural to set a new, even higher goal.

When you look back, however, you may find your partners or associates lagging behind, making no special effort to keep up with you. One explanation: They may not have your drive to achieve. They may be content with their lifestyle and earnings, especially if they're part of a two-income household. Or they may be more interested in pursuing other goals, such as spending more time with their families, or sailing, or whatever. In fact, they may think you're as strange as you think they are.

Accepting that one person's music can be another person's noise can greatly improve the harmony between partners and associates and increase everyone's enjoyment of the practice.

Action Step

Before forming a partnership or taking on an associate, clarify mutual expectations, short- and long-term goals, and what it will take to achieve them. Also draft a letter of your understanding of the arrangement. Doing so won't ensure compliance but it might eliminate the vagueness that can lead to misunderstanding and disappointment.

Not to Decide is to Decide

99

Practice management decisions are seldom easy. Invariably there are arguments both for and against almost any course of action. For example:

- buying new equipment that you don't absolutely need
- firing an employee of long-standing whose work and/or attitude is unsatisfactory
- taking on an associate
- changing your fees
- giving up an enjoyable but unprofitable part of your practice.

Keep in mind that there are very few "perfect" management decisions that are clear-cut choices and by definition, easy to make. The decisions that are 75 percent black and 25 percent white are more common, but still relatively easy to make. Unfortunately, many management decisions fall into the gray, borderline category: 51 percent black, 49 percent white—or vice versa. And those are the toughies.

But as a philosopher once said, "Not to decide is to decide." That statement confronts us with the reality that it's our choice to move forward or stay with the status quo.

If your judgment and experience tell you one of those borderline decisions is the right thing to do, take a leap of faith. Go for it!

As hockey player Wayne Gretzky says, "You miss 100 percent of the shots you don't take."

Will You Have Regrets?

Throughout the years, I've asked countless veterinarians, "What's your single biggest regret in managing your practice?" Among the most common responses:

- **"I didn't spend more time with my family."** Stemming from ambition or dedication—perhaps both—many veterinarians promise their families "not now—later." Doing so results in much borrowing against the future on the assumption there will always be time to be together. But time slips by—and is gone.
- **"I didn't remodel/redecorate my hospital/clinic sooner."** These veterinarians tell me: "I never knew how bad it was until we redecorated and everyone told us how nice it was—and what an improvement it was!"
- **"I didn't raise my fees sooner."** All agreed that client complaints weren't nearly as numerous as they'd feared. Most clients, they said, take reasonable, periodic fee increases in stride; many don't even notice. Even those veterinarians who lost some clients due to fee increases reported an improved overall profitability.

Change is often very difficult to make. Sometimes, however, learning from the experience of others can help you avoid regrets.

100

From the Success File

Deciding to spend more time with his family, a Pennsylvania veterinarian posted this hand-lettered sign in the reception area of his hospital: "Starting January 1st, Daddy's hospital will close at 6 p.m." It was signed "Debby and Billy," his 8- and 10-year-old children. As you might guess, he didn't hear a single complaint.

101

Hard-Learned Lessons about Stress and Other Things That Go Bump in the Night

- No one ever said on his or her deathbed: "I wish I'd spent more time at work."
- A bad partner is worse than no partner.
- In most cases, the things that happen in practice are never as good or bad as they seem at the time.
- Striving for perfection is a blueprint for high-stress living.
- A veterinarian being honest with himself told me: Veterinary medicine didn't cause my mid-life crisis. I did.
- It's not what happens to us but rather our perceptions of what happens that cause almost all forms of emotional stress.
- In a bad situation, you have four options: leave it, change it, accept it, or reframe it. Reframing is a powerful strategy for coping with situations that can't be abandoned or changed and are extremely difficult to accept. Finding a constructive way to look at a situation that gives you a better outlook or a positive personal outcome is the essence of reframing.
- Rules to live by:
    1) Don't sweat the small stuff.
    2) It's all small stuff. (Robert S. Elliot, M.D.)
- For every minute you are angry, you lose one minute of happiness.
- Psychologists say the key to enjoying your work is an

old, nearly forgotten principle: Do your best—not just for the patient and client, but for yourself.

- Rudy Engholm, JD, told me, "Seventy-five percent of my clients could have avoided lawsuits if someone had simply said, 'I'm sorry.'"
- Are hassles with clients about small, long-overdue bills truly worth the time and aggravation of repeated collection efforts or small claims court? If not, consider a year-end greeting card with the following message: "Your unpaid balance of $22 has been forgiven and, as of this date, has been removed from the books. Happy New Year." Some clients will pay what they owe. Others won't. Either way, you're ahead.
- The best thing to save for your old age is yourself.
- The obvious secret: If it is to be, it is up to me.

Notes

Epilogue

Carpe Diem!

At Cornell University, psychologists Thomas Gilovich and Victoria Husted Medvec asked 77 nursing home residents, Cornell students, employees, and professors emeriti to describe the biggest regrets of their lives. Using questionnaires, phone surveys, and one-on-one interviews, they obtained 213 responses.

The results indicate that those surveyed most regret the things in life they failed to do, not the things they did—by a margin of nearly two to one! The most commonly listed regrets? Missed educational opportunities and failures to "seize the moment."

To avoid such regrets, consider the Latin expression "carpe diem," which means seize the day, enjoy the day, or take the opportunity while it is available.

In This Special
Moment in Life

The prologue to this book got you up and running. The epilogue is intended for quiet reflection.

The following paragraph, from a newsletter published by the Interfaith Nutrition Network, of Glen Cove, N.Y., a local soup kitchen, is used with permission:

Think freely. Practice patience. Smile often. Savor special moments. Make new friends. Rediscover old ones. Tell those you love that you do. Feel deeply. Forget trouble. Forgive an enemy. Hope. Grow. Be crazy. Count your blessings. Observe miracles. Let them happen. Discard worry. Give. Give in. Trust enough to take. Pick some flowers. Share them. Keep a promise. Look for rainbows. Gaze at stars. See beauty every-where. Work hard. Be wise. Try to understand. Take time for people. Make time for yourself. Laugh heartily. Spread joy. Take a chance. Reach out. Let someone in. Try something new. Slow down. Be soft sometimes. Believe in yourself. Trust others. See a sunrise. Listen to rain. Reminisce. Cry when you need to. Trust life. Have faith. Enjoy wonder. Comfort a friend. Have good ideas. Make some mistakes. Learn from them. Celebrate life.

Notes

Appendix

A Word to Meeting Planners

Bob Levoy conducts management seminars and workshops for veterinary medical associations, academies, and schools of veterinary medicine.

Bob's speaking style is unique: fast-paced, upbeat, and down-to-earth—with plenty of audience interaction, humor, and most important, practical, immediately usable information.

For further information, contact Bob Levoy at b.levoy@att.net or (516) 626-1353.

Attention Veterinarians and Staff Members: See Your Success Secrets in Print!

If you have a "Success Secret" that would help others build a high-performance practice, please fax or send it to:

> b.levoy@att.net
> or Fax: (516) 626-1340

I'll review it carefully for future use in one of my "Success File" columns in *Veterinary Economics* magazine and/or in a future edition of this book—with, of course, full credit to you.

Note: Your initial submission need be only an overview of the idea. If your Success Secret is selected, I'll get back to you for more details.